gratitude
&grit

A Mother's Healing Journey

by Jacqueline Dunkle

Book Design by Donnia Denig www.donnia.net

ISBN-13: 978-1512157208

ISBN-10: 1512157201

gratitude &grit

A Mother's Healing Journey

Table of Contents

dedication
&thanks

Dedicated to my son, Erik
Wolfgang Fugunt, and all
health care professionals and
healers who make a
difference.

With very special thanks to
New Hanover Regional
Medical Center &
Hospitality House

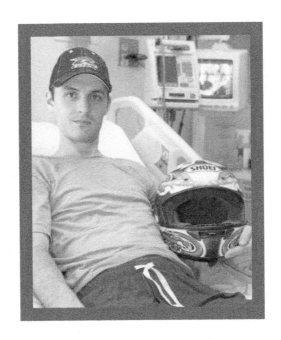

My son, Erik

"Now faith is
the assurance
of things
hoped for,

the conviction
of things
not seen."

Hebrews 11:1

preface

I'd been waiting all my life, for lots of things, but none more dreaded than the news of my son's motorcycle accident. I wonder... how many chances do you get in life? Opportunities to say "hello", "goodnight", "I love you", or "I'm sorry". How many chances do you get in life to live again? To heal wounds, physical and emotional, big and little, known and unknown? I've been given that chance, the chance of a lifetime, the opportunity to say those things again, to heal wounds, to love my son with a deeper awareness and to live my faith in a way I never thought possible. I'm sharing my story with you, with the hope that it might help you live your life, your faith, in ways you never thought possible.

The Call

I'd been waiting for that call for twenty-five years.

Every parent knows the call I'm referring to. It's the one that tells you something tragic has happened to your child; the one that irreversibly changes the course of your life. It was the day that I would receive that call and this is how it began.

It was 11 o'clock in the morning. I looked at the prescription that a doctor had given me for long term thyroid medication. Should I fill it or not? Begrudgingly, I'd already taken a few thyroid pills that were prescribed for me when I collapsed at the Emergency Room three weeks prior. I didn't want to take anymore. Tests confirmed multiple lumps on my thyroid, with a large one visibly protruding from my neck. For the past two months, I'd been struggling with a hyperthyroid. I literally wasn't able to function for more than two hours a day. I'd eat like a horse, then sleep. I had no energy and weight was falling off of me. My body seemed to be eating itself to death. But in my gut, I knew that long term thyroid medication wasn't the solution for me.

I'd researched possible etheric causes of thyroid conditions. The thyroid is associated with the fifth chakra which is responsible for one's ability to communicate. Feeling judged or criticized along with the inability to speak one's truth, can lead to an imbalance in the fifth chakra, therefore

11

an imbalance in the thyroid. My current life situation certainly did reflect feeling judged, criticized and unable to speak my truth. I was silently struggling with personal and professional issues.

I wasn't able to speak my truth regarding both my love relationship and my unconventional career path of Intuitive Healing Coach. My love relationship with Chuck was trying at times, to say the least, due to an unpleasant drawn out divorce. I felt attacked by false accusations about me and my role in his divorce that were made by his estranged family. I did my best to remain silent in the face of those untruths, swallowing the hurt and anger instead of screaming. And I was also having a tough time speaking about the work I'd begun; using intuitive gifts for healing via life coaching. You might say conditions were optimal for a perfect thyroid storm.

So I visited an energy therapist, intuitive medic, nutrition advisor and massage therapist. Each one of those visits enlightened me with even more information to use in my self-healing process. And the visibly protruding lump in my neck shrank to half the size immediately after my first visit with the energy therapist. My belief in natural healing, or at the very least, integrated medicine, was validated and although I didn't feel completely healthy yet, I sensed my energy returning. So I decided to stay the course with natural modalities of healing treatments and tossed the prescription in the garbage.

It was Wednesday, April 14, 2010. I set my intention clearly. Today, I would have more energy. Today, I would get better. Today, I *had* to get better. I started the day slowly, not the least bit aware of how much energy and health would be required of me very soon. It was time to get back into the swing of things, present myself to the world again. Looking back, I try to remember that hour, what I was thinking about, what I was fussing over, what seemed so important during that 11th hour – like checking my emails while coloring my hair. If I'd known what was happening six hundred miles away, my appearance and emails would have meant nothing.

chapter 1 | the call

Pacing myself with a more conscious approach to conserve energy, I went on about my business and left the house to purchase thyroid supplements and then attend an afternoon meeting. As I drove away from the house I remembered that I left my cell phone behind. I decided to keep going without it. What's the worst that can happen? Someone dies? In that case there's nothing I can do anyway. Besides, I'd grown weary of cell phones. They seem to steal our sense of presence. We aren't designed to be available around the clock. So leaving my cell phone behind certainly wasn't the end of the world but it did set the scene for a desperate search that day. Around 4 o'clock, I was in the midst of that afternoon meeting when, my friend, Mandy unexpectedly appeared. I was surprised to see her and simply thought she wanted to see the facility that I'd been consulting with. I excitedly began to show her around when she asked, "Have you talked to Chuckie? He's trying to reach you."

I had been active for about five hours by now and my energy was holding steady. "Oh, he's such a worry wart!" I blew her off completely. "He's working out of town in Memphis and I left my cell phone at the house. He's probably worried because I've been so weak and he can't reach me. He'll be fine!" I continued on with no clue to the real reason she was there. As we walked on, Mandy gently touched my arm and said, "I *really* think you need to call Chuckie."

This time I stopped walking. "Is everything okay?" I asked, furrowing my brow a bit. She handed me her phone and had already dialed his number. "Just call him." Alright, she had my attention now. I could feel the heat rise in my body. It wasn't full blown panic yet, but certainly heightened concern. Chuck, my future husband, answered the phone. "Hello?" He answered with anxiety and hesitation, expecting to hear Mandy's voice because it was Mandy's phone. "Honey, it's me, Jacq. Is everything okay?" My heightened concern was morphing into an adrenaline rush.

"No." He replied with a gentle firm tone, then a pause. "Erik's been in an accident ... on his motorcycle."

I closed my eyes and took a very deep breath. Because of my ex-husband and son's adventurous lifestyle, I'd been waiting and preparing myself for that phone call for twenty-five years; expecting it to arrive sooner or later. My son, Erik and I had talked about it many times, the most recent being 11 months prior when my best friend's son, Bubba, was killed in an accident. As I sobbed, I told Erik that I always thought it would be me that would get that phone call; that my son had been killed in an accident, not my best friend's son, Bubba; he wasn't the daredevil. Erik agreed with me and couldn't explain his many near escapes or why he was still alive. But he assured me that he was at peace with dying and not afraid, so whatever happened, he wanted me to be okay and know that he was alright. He said, "If I go before you do, you'll always feel me when you're near the water. You know I love the sea." Maybe that's not something all moms and sons discuss, but I'm glad we did, because the dreaded moment had arrived. I hadn't dodged the bullet after all. This was the call that I knew would eventually come. The weakening rush of adrenaline was taking over my body. I sat down on the floor, back against the wall and put my head between my legs, forcing myself to ask Chuck the mother lode of all questions, "Is he still alive?"

Time was suspended in the second that it took Chuck to answer me. I can't imagine how hard it was for him to speak or what he must have been going through as he frantically tried to locate me. He'd been contacted by my ex-husband, Ron, who couldn't reach me. Chuck then contacted my friend, Mandy, who physically searched the town and hunted me down because he couldn't reach me by phone. Of all days to rid myself of that cell phone, I had to pick this one. *What's the worst that could happen? Someone dies? And if that happened, there would be nothing I could do anyway.* I wanted to choke on my thoughts.

Chuck answered hesitantly, "Yes, he's – still alive." Sensing from the way he answered, I already knew the answer to my next question, but asked it anyway. "How bad is it?"

"It's pretty bad." He replied. I knew from the tone of his voice that this was a crossroads of life and death. Chuck has an incredibly soft heart so I knew he threw the word "pretty" in there to soften the blow of bad news. I knew instinctively that it was more than pretty bad. It was bad, very bad, the worst. I'd heard all that I needed to hear. "I'm on my way. I'll meet you there. Goodbye Chuck." I spoke so directly it almost felt like an order. I suppose it was an order; a battle order. The battle of the crossroads between life and death had begun. And I was up for the fight of my life; the fight for my son's life.

When Erik's father and I divorced, emotions and circumstances were so volatile that I proposed joint custody and didn't fight for primary care of Erik. I also didn't want to drag my son through the experience of an ugly custody battle. It was a horribly difficult decision to make. It haunted me for seventeen years. And even though we had joint custody, many of my ex-relatives took the stance that I had abandoned my son. There was much anguish that accompanied my decision. How would it affect my son's perspective of women, his trust? Nonetheless, I felt it was safest and best for everyone, not to fight. That was seventeen years ago. This was now. This time would be different. This time, I'd go to my grave fighting for my son. This time my ex-husband and I would fight, in unison.

I departed quickly from the meeting, in an urgent flurry of disbelief, tears suspended in my eyes. Mandy followed me as I rushed home and assisted me in the most efficiently orchestrated exodus I'd ever known. While I tossed some clothes in a bag, she checked flights from Pittsburgh, Pennsylvania to Wilmington, North Carolina.

I called Ron, my ex-husband. He sounded completely distraught and forlorn, which confirmed it was as bad as I'd thought. "It's not good, Jacq." His voice quivered. "They don't know if he'll live. And if he does pull through, they say he'll be paralyzed. He won't want to live like that Jacq, not if he can't walk. I know him. He won't want to live like that."

Ron and I had divorced seventeen years ago and had since settled our differences. I felt his despair and loss. We shared the same child and the same love for that child, "It'll be okay," I said. "It'll be okay, Ron." I was acting like a boxing coach, psyching up a scrappy middle weight fighter who had just gotten the snot kicked out of him. I knew sentimentality and sympathy wouldn't help any of us at this point. He needed something to help him, help Erik. Aside from loving them both, I lived with them for ten action packed years, witnessing stunts galore from their activities of boating, horseback riding, hang gliding, motorcycling, hunting, fishing, diving and flying small planes. Believe me; the list goes on and on. And I'm sure I'd only seen a fraction of what they'd done to try and one-up the other. I knew this daredevil duo pretty well. I knew their temperaments; I knew of their conversations about "offing" the other if something tragic ever happened. "It'll be okay Ron," I continued with a steady voice. "Let's just get him through this. He loves being on two wheels so much, he'll just have two strapped to his ass permanently if he can't walk. Hang on. I'm on my way. I'll be there sometime late tonight."

I hung up with Ron when Chuck called to check the progress of travel arrangements. He was leaving Memphis and flying to Wilmington. It would take him about six hours to get there, so he'd be there before me. Mandy had determined that I'd never make it to the airport in time for the last flight out of Pittsburgh, especially with Penguin hockey traffic. As usual, Mandy thought of everything. Driving to Wilmington was the solution. "Jacq, I really don't want you driving." Chuck pleaded. "Please wait until morning and fly down."

"Chuck," my voice was sharp and stern, "If your son was lying in a hospital and you may have one chance to see him before he died, would you wait until morning? This is *not* open for discussion. Goodbye. I love you. I'll see you there." He conceded. "Jacq, please be careful. I love you. And I need you. Please be safe."

I grabbed my tossed bag of clothes and thyroid supplements, jumped in the car, waved to Mandy and sped off. A few miles down the road, the first call I made was to my mother. She answered in her usual chipper way and I quickly cut to the chase. "Mama, I have some sad news. Erik's been in a motorcycle accident. It's bad. We don't know if he's going to make it. I'm driving to North Carolina as we speak and I need you to have Dad call me with directions. I don't want to waste time to stop and look at the map. I think I remember the way, but I need to make sure. Oh Mama, please pray. Please pray."

Like always, the sound of her loving voice fueled my strength, faith and resolve. My mom is a pillar. "Oh honey, of course we will pray without ceasing. Oh Jacque, you've been so weak with your thyroid. I'm so concerned about you. Are you okay to drive?" My mother's concern was warranted as she had seen me a few weeks ago when I could barely stand.

"Yep Mom, I'm good. I feel strong." Even to my own surprise, I really was feeling strong enough to handle it; adrenaline, I guess. "Just have Dad call me as soon as he can, please." My father was out on the farm somewhere but Mom assured me that she'd find him and get him back to the house. Our family dynamics resembled that of an Amish family, only with electricity. My parents raised me and my three older siblings on a farm in Frogtown, Pennsylvania. So I had been exposed to the natural life cycles of animals and crops my entire life. That upbringing coupled with consistent church activities fostered a deep faith within our almost Amish family; a faith that sustained us through many difficult times.

But we'd never faced a time like this. My parents were in their seventies and still had every child, grandchild, and great-grandchild intact with no lives lost. It looked like that would all change now. We hung up with Mom instructing me to be careful. Don't we all say that? You know, I could have called anyone for directions. So the call to home was all about needing their love and support, not directions. It was just a good cover since my father was not only a farmer but also a lifetime truck driver that knew highways and interstates like the back of his hand. Dad knew me like the back of his hand too.

My phone showed numerous missed calls from Lori. She must know about the accident. Oh God, how is she going to process this? We'd been best friends for nearly twenty years and she now owned the spa – an adventure we started out on together – a business I once owned and sold to her. Exactly 11 months ago, her eighteen year old son, Michael "Bubba", was killed in a tragic accident in which he was thrown from the back of a pickup truck.

Oh God, I had to call her. What would I say? My heart reminded me that no words were necessary. We'd been friends through thick and thin for so long. I hit her speed dial. Her voice was just what I expected, grievous yet powerful and courageous. She wanted to ride to North Carolina with me but I told her that I wasn't slowing down for anything. I needed to get there. I needed to see him. As much as she wanted to be with me, she completely understood, like no one else could. She'd been in those shoes, frantically searching for her son in a hospital when she got word that he had been in an accident. She never found him at a hospital. He'd been pronounced dead at the scene. "Dear God, how much more can we take?" she asked. "What the hell is going on?" This could not be happening. Not to both of us. Not best friends. Not this close together. What was God trying to tell us? This just couldn't be real. But it was real. Very real. We signed off, knowing that each would be there for the other. Like always, she was my Rock.

Armored with love from Chuck, faith from Mama, and power from Lori, I gathered up all the hope I could find within me and headed for the front lines on the battlefield that awaited me many miles ahead at New Hanover Regional Medical Center in Wilmington, North Carolina. "I'm coming Erik," I whispered. "Hold on, honey. I'm coming."

Then I began to sing a lovely hymn that I learned as a child and sang whenever I needed comforted at a place too deep to describe. It seems the writer of this hymn, Horatio Spafford had suffered tremendous losses of his own. First, he lost his real estate fortune in the devastating Great Chicago Fire. Two years later, in 1873 he sent his wife and four daughters on a ship ahead of him to Europe for a vacation. All four of his daughters died in a fateful ship wreck on route and only the mother survived, rescued from a floating plank, to arrive in England. Mr. Spafford immediately went to his wife in England and reportedly wrote the hymn, *It Is Well With My Soul* as he sailed over the precise location of his daughters' deaths. Now I understand why this hymn comforts me. The personal experience of horrendous human loss soothed by Christ's divine peace is intimately lodged in his words and will touch any soul that is open to its message.

When peace, like a river, attendeth my way,
When sorrows like sea billows roll,
Whatever my lot, Thou hast taught me to say,
It is well, it is well with my soul.

It is well (it is well) with my soul (with my soul)
It is well; it is well with my soul.

For me, be it Christ, be it Christ hence to live,
If Jordan above me shall roll,
No pain shall be mine, for in death as in life,
Thou wilt whisper Thy peace to my soul.

The Driving Force

So what do you do while driving six hundred miles, unsure of what you will find when you arrive at the Intensive Care Trauma Unit that is harboring your child? Would Erik be alive? Would he be dead? Would he be mangled? Would he be paralyzed? Would he be able to hear me? Would he *ever* be able to hear, see or know anyone again?

Hung in the balance of life and death, time started to disappear. Actually, an awful lot disappeared. Gone were the concerns of my health, my work, my relationships, of money, of schedules and unnecessary drama.

Gone were the concerns of everything, everything but seeing and touching Erik's face.

I knew whatever outcome that awaited me at that hospital, I had been altered and that life as I'd known it was over. Everything was different now. Everything.

I called the hospital where Erik lie waiting. I left my number and a message with ICU that I was on my way. Not long after, a woman named Louise called me back. She was the ICU nurse that was attending to Erik. She calmly conveyed that Erik was alive and that he was somehow holding his own for now. I asked her to *please* tell Erik something for me. She agreed.

"Please whisper in his ear that Mama's coming... (I started to sob)... and that Trixie is right there with him."

"Trixie?" Louise questioned me.

"Yes," I said, "That's the name he gave his guardian angel and she must be with him overtime today."

"I'll tell him," she promised. "Now, you drive carefully and I'll see you when you get here." And we hung up.

Then something shifted. Suddenly, there was no such thing as time. There was only now, only presence. I was unusually comforted in a way that I can't describe. It felt as though I was suspended in God's time. In the midst of this heart wrenching, painful situation, there was a peace invisibly floating up through me like smoke from a fire. I knew it was there, I just couldn't see it or capture it, but I could feel it. The fire burning inside of me was the pain and the suffering in my soul. I had to let myself *feel* it. I had to let it burn. It was the only way the smoke of peace would come; that place of grace – that place of God. I've read that suffering has a mystical transformative power. Indeed, it does.

So as I drove, I wept. You know when you're driving, and you look at other people driving, and they're doing something like singing with the music, or picking their nose? I actually wondered as I was driving, how many people I'd ever seen bawling. If anyone looked over at me, they'd have seen me bawling and known I was suffering.

Tears streamed down my pitiful face like a river. As I wept, I spoke to Erik in spirit. I told him how much I loved him. I told him that he was a wonderful, kind young man. I told him he was always destined to be my pride and joy. I told him that I learned so much about life from him. I told him I was sorry that I didn't keep him safe. I told him that even though I divorced his father, I always loved him. I told him that we shared a mystical and divine connection that nothing could destroy – not even death. I told him that I understood if he had to go. I told him that I was selfish and asked him to stay. I told him that it was his life – his choice to stay or go. I told him that I would honor his choice. And I wept. I wondered if this was the "exit" he was going to take and I wondered why he would want to take it. His life had taken such a hopeful change of direction in the past three months with the choices he'd made; returning to Cape Fear Community College and to his big surprise, loving it; meeting a lovely young woman and believing in love again after a difficult split with a former girlfriend of five years. I spoke out loud, all of these things, to Erik.

As a steady stream of tears fell, they dripped upon and dampened the painful, burning fire inside, creating more smoke of peace that filled me, so that I would suddenly stop sobbing and be completely present with it all. Those were the sober moments when I received and made calls to family and friends; when I matter-of-factly cancelled my travel plans to Dallas for the weekend to see my sister and nieces, when I called my friend Michele, a nurse who had worked extensively with spinal cord injury patients. I left a message on her cell phone with complete composure and clarity, "Michele. It's Jacque. My son, Erik has been in a motorcycle accident. I'm in my car, on my way to North Carolina right now and I don't know if he'll be dead or alive when I arrive. I'm told that if he lives, he'll be paralyzed. I want you to prepare me for what I'm going to see. Love you." She returned my call within the hour. "Does he have a head trauma?" she asked. I hadn't been told of any head trauma at this point. "If he doesn't have head trauma, you'll be okay. You can do this," she assured me. "If he does have head trauma, it's a whole different ball game. Let's just hope and pray that he doesn't. Travel safely. And I love you, Sister." We weren't blood sisters but we were "sisters". I trusted Michele's expertise and knew she would be truthful with me, no matter what. That conversation helped me focus on "doing this" as I drove 80 mph across the Pennsylvania turnpike.

My composure was somewhat intact until the phone began to ring like croaking frogs. It's the selected ringtone for my parents who live in Frogtown. Mom had found my father. He was calling with directions. My heart skipped a beat. As much as I wanted to hear his voice, I knew that when I did hear it, I'd want to cry. I took a deep breath, exhaled, and then answered with teetering composure, "Hi Dad."

"Jacque, are you okay?" Somehow, with quivering voices we both managed to keep it together, trying not to fall apart for the sake of the other. We focused on the best possible driving routes and then I would repeat them back to Dad to help me memorize them. I could always count on my father for direction. Ask anyone. He's good at giving it! Admittedly, many times I don't listen. But this time, I listened. I listened very closely. I hung on each resonating tone of his voice. Just as Mama's voice provided me with strength and resolve, Dad's voice provided me with serenity and clarity. Road maps can't do that; my father can. We choked back our tears as we said goodbye. His direction and focus were embedded in my mind.

I wondered if anyone had called Erik's girlfriend, Jenny. I hadn't met her yet. They had only been dating for about six weeks, but Erik had a deep respect for her and was filled with tenderness when he spoke of her. I sensed that love was growing for them and I believed her presence would have a powerful impact on his will to live. God, I hoped someone knew how to get in touch with her. God, I hoped she was there. I didn't know she was already there. She and Erik had planned a trip to Florida and were scheduled to leave that afternoon when Jenny got the call from Erik's little brother, Nick. She was pumping gas preparing for her three hour drive to Wilmington from Mebane. Needless to say, her three hour drive took much less time. She arrived midafternoon and faithfully stayed by Erik's side.

I was cruising along at a pretty good clip, making great time, when my Aunt Carol called. I had just spoken with her daughter, my cousin, Ronda Kay, about Erik's accident. Word travels fast. Carol asked that I stop to pick her up so she could help drive. Carol was just six years older than me so she was more like a big sister than an aunt. She lived just a few miles from I95, the interstate that I was traveling but I was determined not to waste any time stopping for anything but fuel. I declined her offer to help drive. But she was persistent and wouldn't take no for an answer.

Man, I just wanted to get there! Being alone was comfortable for me. I could bawl and not have anyone see me; and the need to concentrate on my task of driving kept me from falling apart. I *really* didn't want to stop. I was agitated that I'd agreed to it. So help me God, if Erik wasn't alive by the time I got there...oh man, I'd never forgive myself.

Honestly though, stopping for Carol was a good thing. She always was naturally calming, not one to get overly excited about things, with the exception being Pittsburgh Steelers football. We talked about other things to help pass the time. I received and made a lot of phone calls. I saved many messages that were left on my voicemail by family and friends; messages of love, prayers and support; messages that comfort me still to this day when I listen to them again.

When we got within fifty miles, I felt my stomach getting sick. I put my head between my knees. Then Chuck's ID picture appeared on the front of my cell phone as it rang. Why was he calling now? I'm almost there! Oh God, please don't tell me that Erik is dead. Please don't tell me that I didn't make it in time. I answered the phone frantically, "Is he still alive?"

As planned, Chuck had arrived before me and found his way to Erik. "Yes, he's still alive. And Jacq, he's not mangled. On the outside, he doesn't look that bad. Ron and I will meet you at the night entrance of the Trauma ICU." Erik's commitment to wearing full riding gear paid off by protecting his appearance, but internally speaking, there is only so much gear you can wear for protection.

It wouldn't be long now, until I could see him, touch him. Just breathe. Breathe deeply. Breathe again. Keep breathing. I was almost there. I wasn't sure if I was breathing for me or for Erik. I'm guessing both.

It seemed the closer we got, the slower Carol drove. It was about 1 a.m. when we pulled into the hospital parking. Could she go any slower? Man, it took everything I had not to jump out of that car and run through the hospital doors, run to my son. I struggled to stay cool and composed. I waited until she parked to scramble from the car. Confident, deliberate steps carried me to the night entrance where Ron, my ex-husband, and Chuck, my future husband, were waiting.

While Chuck and Carol quietly spoke, I tearfully hugged Ron, squeezed his hand and said, "Come on. We can do this. We'll get through this." Down the long hallway to the ICU we marched. The front battle line was just ahead. Chuck was the perfect handler; close enough to hold us up, far enough to observe and anticipate our needs. He picked up the phone that was used to keep the ICU secure and asked for permission to enter.

Are you kidding me? I need permission to enter? I was ready to storm the doors that stood between me and my son. Come on! Open the damn door! Breathe. Breathe deeply.

Click. The door opened. Indeed, the door opened. Knock and the door shall be opened unto you. The door to Erik, the door to life, the door to death, the door to healing, the door to love, they all opened; a door that would never be closed again.

ICU aka I See You

Chuck and Ron led the way through the Intensive Care Unit and I took Carol's hand as we approached Room 8. Erik was in that room, behind the drawn privacy curtain. "You can do this," Carol assured me. I squeezed her hand and nodded my head. She didn't let on but told me later that she felt faint. Sure, I could do this, while she passed out beside me. But she didn't pass out. And I prayed silently, "Grace me with strength, dear God. Grace me with strength." My chest lifted with yet another deep breath and my heart felt as though it would explode as my legs carried me boldly to the front line of battle. Nothing could stop me now. I felt the armor and power of God's love surround me. I stepped inside the room. And there it was - his face.

I saw my son's amazing face. Amazing Face, Amazing Grace.

They were
synonymous now.

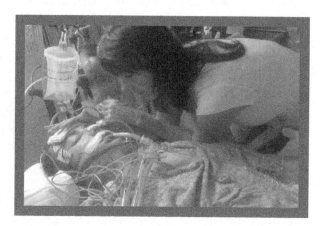

Erik, I see you

Amidst all the tubes, wires, beeping monitors and repetitive puffs of the respirator, I felt the presence of God; I was transported to a Secret Garden of Grace, the most sacred place I've ever experienced. Bending close to his ear, I quietly spoke to my only child. "Mama's here now, Baby. Everything's gonna be okay. Just rest now. And believe. Know that you are so very loved. Know that you are the most important thing. Know that you matter so much. Everything's gonna be okay. You're gonna be okay. I love you Erik. I love you so much." The words stopped and gave way to a delicate shower of kisses with special ones strategically placed directly on his third eye chakra and at the inner corners of his eyes; the same places I would caress and kiss him when he was a baby.

Eventually, I was able to step back and observe the rest of his body. I saw that everyone I'd mentioned before was still in the room. They weren't gone. It was me who had left to enter the Secret Garden and walk there with my son. I thought of my grandmother's favorite hymn, *In the Garden*, and began to hum it quietly as I carefully inspected the rest of his body.

Because of extensive emergency surgery on his lungs, Erik was connected to an oscillating respirator that was used for infants. It continually pumped one hundred baby breaths per minute into his lungs; enough pressure to keep them inflated but gentle enough to keep the stitches in his lung from tearing, hopefully. It shook his entire body like a muffled jack hammer. He looked like a robot human hybrid under construction. No accident or trauma care wounds were visible to me yet except for a small red mark on his left hand. His body was swelled considerably and seemed to continue to swell in front of our eyes.

I scanned him slowly from head to toe. When I reached his feet, I was fixated like a laser. I stood at the foot of his bed and kissed his feet and cried, then kissed his feet some more. As my tears fell onto his feet, I would massage them into his skin. I suddenly felt like the queen Mary Magdalene, adorning her Lord's feet with anointed oils. My oils were my tears. I kissed each perfect toe, one by one, a ritual I continued for days to come. If only my tears were as holy as the Christ's, maybe my son would live, maybe my son would walk.

After a few hours I had filled Erik and myself completely with adoring love. I was able to gather my wits and meet Louise, the wonderful woman who'd been caring for Erik since he first made it to ICU.

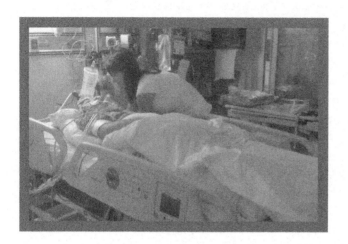

Erik, ICU

If we were in the Secret Garden, Louise would have been the biggest sunflower I'd ever seen. Her smile was so bright and cheerful. She effortlessly managed to transform all that happy energy into highly focused and skilled ICU nursing care. I asked if she had whispered in his ear, the message that "Mama's coming and Trixie is with you." She grinned and said, "Yes, but I did look around first, to see if anyone was watching. I didn't want to look crazy." She giggled a bit. Again, only Louise could pull off a giggle in the middle of this highly charged, traumatic and deeply emotional moment of life and death.

I could sense that Louise was a woman of faith. The way she delivered it was so sunny and refreshing. I immediately trusted her and confided in her about my own health, to help ensure that my physical strength would hold up considering my thyroid condition.

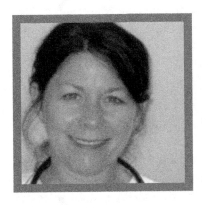

My ICU Sunshine,
Louise,
aka Weezie

*Photo Courtesy of New
Regional Medical*

Conveying my preferences for holistic treatment, she recommended a local pharmacy that specialized in natural supplements as well as pharmaceuticals. She also noticed that I used stones when I prayed over Erik, so she told me of a local place where I could get stones and oils as well. I placed my pale green healing stone that had a reiki symbol naturally embedded in it on Erik's chest, between his toes and on his third eye, consistently throughout the hospital stay. Louise was not only an excellent ICU nurse, she was also a divine messenger and I have no doubt that she is fulfilling God's purpose for her life, perfectly. Even now when I think of her, I see a sky full of sunshine coming from her soul. And I can't think of a place that needs sunshine more than an ICU.

I spent the wee hours of that night at Erik's bedside, with the exception of a few moments outside his room, talking with his attending physician. Since I was well aware of the gravity of the situation, I had a lingering sense of duty to ask the heavy dreaded question. "Doctor," I asked directly, "Is my son considered *on life support*? Because if that's the case, I know his wishes and his father and I will make the necessary decision to carry them out. Is it time for us to make that decision?" I couldn't believe what I was actually saying. I was prepared to pull the proverbial plug. My tear-streaked face was serious, distraught and pitiful, I'm sure.

"Absolutely not!" the doctor responded firmly and quickly. "He's made it this far. We have to see what happens. It's not time for that, no way." I was convinced, but deep down, I wondered if that's just what doctors said after they'd invested so much into keeping their patients alive. At that point, I didn't realize what Erik had already come through, what they had already witnessed fourteen hours ago and throughout the day. It seemed as though my son was up to his usual tricks of shocking people; this time by surviving the past fourteen hours. Maybe that's why he named his guardian angel Trixie.

He'd just shocked the heck out of everyone in the Emergency Room and ICU with his strength, spirit and will to survive. Why should I be surprised? He'd been shocking me for years. He's my only child, my pride and joy. I just never expected anyone else to see it. But by now, a lot of people were seeing it. At noon on Thursday, April 15th, standing by Erik's bedside, Chuck and I hugged one another. Erik had made it through twenty-four hours. Let's try for another twenty-four, another day to love and be loved.

Injuries & Angels

The Webster Dictionary definition of a miracle is this: ***an extraordinary event manifesting divine intervention in human affairs.*** I'll share the facts. You decide for yourself if there were miracles in the making on the morning of April 14, 2010.

Within a minute of Erik's impact with the tree, he was surrounded by people of faith. A man driving by the scene of the accident realized what had just happened. He immediately called 911 and stopped as Erik was motionless except for a feeble fumbling attempt to remove his helmet. That man, Rick, held Erik's head and calmly spoke with him, encouraging him to be still until the EMT arrived. Erik didn't speak. His only response was a dim stare.

The neighbors that lived nearby also ran to Erik's side immediately after the impact. A husband and wife, Don and Kay, were people with deep capacity to share God's love. They stayed with Erik during those early moments and created a circle of prayer along with a woman that witnessed the accident and returned to the scene. The EMS response team of firemen and paramedics were dispatched at 11:23 a.m. They arrived on the scene at 11:30 a.m. and worked expediently to remove his helmet and cut away his riding gear. After a rapid first aid response and assessment, one of the paramedics was heard to say, "We gotta go. I mean NOW!" Erik was in route to the hospital just eight minutes after their arrival. On the way to the hospital, the EMS responders worked feverishly to keep Erik alive. They called to him, "Erik...Erik!" attempting to keep eye contact, which was fading along with his vital signs. He wasn't responding to their efforts. There was blood coming from his nose and mouth. All I know is that I was told he presented with a zero percent chance of survival upon arrival to the hospital at 11:47 a.m. The trauma team at the Emergency Trauma Bay was activated and ready when he arrived. He was clinically dead and unresponsive. He wasn't breathing. They were losing him. The trauma team continued to work on Erik. Again, all their efforts to resuscitate him failed. Half of the trauma team voted to call it quits and let Erik go. The other half voted to keep trying. Doctor Mindy, a fourth year resident, and Bill, the respiratory guy, were the major players that voted to keep fighting for Erik's life.

Not until early Sunday morning, five days after the crash, did I have the opportunity to speak with them about what happened in the Emergency Trauma Bay. Doctor Mindy began to brief me on Erik's condition in the ICU. His left chest and side was stapled shut from an extensive emergency lung surgery. The tracheotomy and ventilator would be required for quite some time, until his lungs proved he could breathe on his own. His heart was bruised, likely from the constant CPR. His left scapula was broken. His shoulder was badly bruised. His pelvis was broken. He was swelling up everywhere, partly from the trauma and partly from fluids being administered. And his T9 vertebra was not only shattered but a fragment of bone was wedged into his spinal column, causing the paralysis. She was amazed, to say the least, that he had made it thus far. Everyone was. She firmly and cautiously warned me that we were not *out of the woods* by any means. She explained that moving forward every decision about treatment would require finding a balance between benefit versus risk. I asked her if she would tell me what happened in the ER the day my son arrived. "Are you sure you want to hear?" she winced.

"Yes." I replied. So she began her story. She was on rounds somewhere in the hospital when her pager sounded and flashed the code of *1111*. Well unbeknownst to her, *1111* was my favorite number so instead of having me at "hello" she had me at "*1111*".

That was the code used to beckon her immediately to the ER Trauma Unit where she would meet an unresponsive young man named Erik.

The respiratory guy, Bill, was trying to intubate Erik's lungs but it wasn't working. So they poked holes into his sides to determine why his lungs wouldn't hold oxygen but they still couldn't detect the problem. Time was running out, and maybe already had run out. They feared his brain had been without oxygen for too long. So even if they could pull off a miracle and resuscitate him, he'd have brain damage.

That's when half voted to quit. But half decided to keep trying; the half of Bill and Doctor Mindy. They looked at each other and a moment of perfect clarity came over them. The fourth year resident, Doctor Mindy boldly reached her finger into the exploratory hole they had poked into his left side and tore his ribcage away from the lining of his lungs. With that one courageous move, ungodly amounts of blood poured from Erik's chest as fast as it was being administered and he bled out on the table.

They quickly rough cut his left side open only to have his left lung fall out in pieces. It had been shredded by the sharp edges of eight completely broken ribs. No wonder he wasn't breathing. Bill had been intubation the left lung which was now just a shredded organ unable to hold anything. He quickly switched to the right lung to intubate Erik. Doctor Mindy reached into Erik's chest and grabbed his heart. Feeling blood still in the chambers, she grabbed all the major vessels and pressed them against his spine as they literally ran down the hall with her hands in his chest, clutching his heart for dear life. They burst unannounced into an empty emergency surgical room where a specialized respiratory surgeon, who just happen to be on call that morning, stitched his lungs back together like folds on a baseball.

I sat there for a few moments, stunned, just gazing at Doctor Mindy. Finally I responded with piercing curiosity and asked,

"What made you
  reach into
  that hole and
  tear his ribcage
  away from his
  lungs?

What made you do it,
when everyone
  else had given up?"

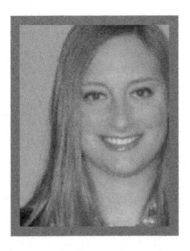

Doctor Mindy

Photo courtesy of
New Hanover Regional
Medical Center

Her answer said it all,
"Intuition."

This lovely, unassuming young woman, held my son's heart in her hands, literally and figuratively. The left side of his body, his feminine side, was destroyed; yet his heart was being firmly held by a young woman refusing to let him go, a young woman fighting for his life. She was about the same age that I was when Erik's father and I divorced and I chose not to fight over who would gain primary care. From my perspective, the coincidences were unbelievable. She fought for Erik's life in ways that I couldn't. She held Erik's heart in a way that I couldn't. We'd been shot back to a time in need of much healing, the time of the divorce in which the female didn't fight.

Well, if the Sacred Feminine was biding her time, waiting to the perfect moment to fight, she'd picked a doozey of a perfect moment.

I smiled softly. I thanked her, then reached to touch her and said, "Always listen to your intuition. I think you know there is much more going on here than meets the eye. *1111* has been my favorite number since I was nine years old. I believe we are all connected and that you were here as part of a divine purpose to save Erik's life by getting that number on your pager." I told her of how Erik's former girlfriend broke up with him on *11:11* and how he'd been seeing that number constantly during the month before the accident and that the girl he'd recently fallen in love with was born on *11:11*. As I spoke with Doctor Mindy about the serendipitous and miraculous events that she had been part of, tears began to form in her eyes. I thought she was tearing up because she was moved by my story, but I was the one surprised when she spoke. "My father died on *11:11.*"

The look coming through her eyes told me that her father's guiding hand was with her that day, telling her what to do, so that my son might live. Thank you, Mindy. Thank you, Mindy's Dad. I held her hands. Our tearful smiles needed no translation.

Jason, a friend of Erik's, made a unique present for Erik to give to Doctor Mindy so she'd never forget how much she meant to all of us. He handcrafted an exquisite sculpture; a lovely flower made of steel, growing from stone; a symbolic gift of our *Gratitude* for her *Grit*; the perfect cover for this book.

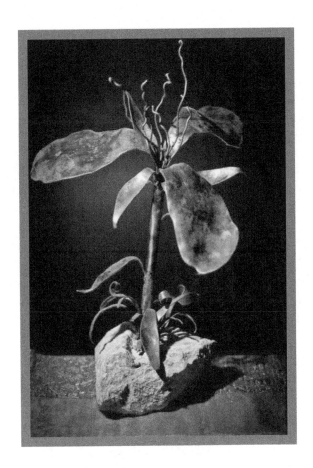

The Love Story

The first time I saw Jenny was in the lounge of the ICU the night I arrived. She was curled up and sleeping on a love seat. She fit perfectly, all ninety pounds of her. Because of the way he spoke of her, I knew with all my heart that her presence would be the deciding factor for Erik's will to survive.

You see, Chuck and I made an impromptu visit to see Erik about three weeks before the accident. I just felt the need to go. Thank God I trusted my intuition. We went and had a great time. Erik even took me for a bike ride in the parking lot before we left. We talked a lot about Jenny the entire weekend. It was obvious that Erik was completely taken with her. During lunch, every conversation wound its way back to her name. We also had a short conversation with a stranger in the restaurant before we left, about helmets. He was a man from Ireland who was visiting America.

Me with Erik
March 2010

three weeks prior
to the accident

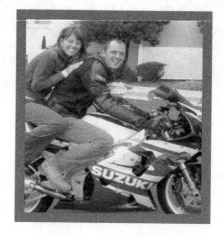

He gestured to Erik's helmet as he approached our table then asked him why so many people here did not wear helmets when they rode motorcycle. Erik smiled, "I don't know," he replied. "I wear one. My head's worth protecting!" Erik *always* wore a good helmet. That's one thing he never skimped on. It makes me wonder sometimes, if maybe on some level, he knew his fate.

But that day, none of us consciously knew how soon that helmet would be doing its job of protecting Erik's head. As we departed, Chuck said, "Please, Erik. Be careful."

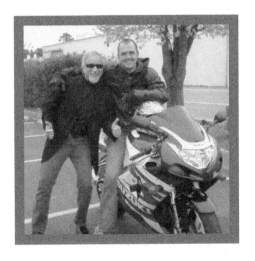

Chuck with Erik

March 2010

"I will," Erik smiled that charming smile. We hugged him goodbye, never imagining that the next time we'd see him, he wouldn't be seeing us and we'd be in the ICU of New Hanover Regional Medical Center.

About ten years prior, Erik had met Jenny in high school. They never really dated, just hung out for a brief period of time before each of them went their own way in the world. That was until two months ago when Jenny had a dream about Erik and decided to look him up on Facebook. What she found was Erik on guard, because his former girlfriend of five years had broken up with him. He's a faithful guy by nature. His loyalty was so thick, that it might be called stubbornness at times. That breakup was on 11:11, November 11, 2009 and Erik didn't take it so well. He called me to talk about it. I told him that 11:11 had been my favorite number since I was a little girl and that it was an opening for a whole new life for him. Even though it hurt and made no sense to him, it would be okay, even better than okay if he focused on positive things, what was important to him in life and asserted himself to take action. It was an emotional blow but he was finding his way through it.

Erik's Facebook (one month before the accident)

Erik Fugunt

The best part of being single is finding the perfect partner all over again!

March 11, 2010 at 8:30pm

Erik Fugunt

Everything happens for a reason and when that reason reveals itself you can't help but stand in

March 22, 2010 at 10:00am

As fate would have it, after finding him on Facebook, Jenny and Erik began to date. He spoke so highly of her – intelligent, mature, strong, fun, independent and fiery. I was so happy for him. I knew how badly he wanted a family and home.

He'd always told me all he really ever wanted was a family and a simple life full of love. And I wished that for him, more than anything. I knew that Erik was brilliant and had so much to offer, but also had a lot of growing up to do and it seemed as though that may be happening. He was becoming such a mature and focused young man. Most importantly, *he* was realizing how much he had to offer; excelling in his college courses, experiencing new people in his life and taking a chance on love again.

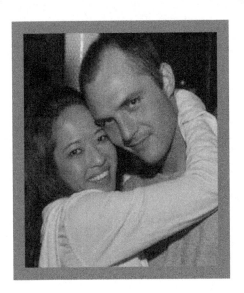

Jenny and Erik

Azalea Festival in Wilmington NC

just days before the accident

Now, here is where it gets even crazier. Ten days before the accident, I received this text from Erik:

> *Moma,*
> *Jenny's bday is*
> *1111. What does*
> *that mean?*
> *And every time I*
> *call or think of her*
> *its 1111 or 111.*
> *So any ideas?*

> *Cool! My favorite*
> *numbers! So 1111 is a*
> *gateway to a life you*
> *create with ur conscious*
> *intention. Also a number*
> *that God's lightworkers*
> *identify with. A portal for*
> *your life path is opening!*
> *Stay the course and*
> *embrace Erikness!*
> *- Moma*

So when I first met Jenny in the waiting room, I already had an idea that she was no ordinary young woman. Her relationship with Erik was part of a divine path. I hugged her and thanked her for being there. Chuck had already preempted the situation before I had arrived. He spoke with Jenny and told her that it was okay if she wanted to go. Since she and Erik had only dated a short time we really didn't expect her to stay.

"I'm not going anywhere!" she held her ground emphatically. "I love him. This is where I want to be."

Wow, huh? I knew it. I just knew it. With that statement, Chuck instantly claimed Jenny as one of our own. And he knew I would as well. Jenny stayed around the clock for five days. Her parents, Chinese immigrants, came to be with us too. It was difficult for me to understand her father's words but her mother spoke more clearly.

Jenny's mother told me that it didn't matter if Erik had a lot of money or a big fancy house. What mattered was that her Jenny loved him and that he made her happy. The voice coming from her petite body spoke with wisdom and intense strength, "Tell him to fight. Whisper it in his ear. Fight Erik. Fight for your life, because you are."

Coincidentally, Erik's former girlfriend was also Chinese and we knew from that experience that he didn't exactly fit the mold as a husband for a Chinese daughter. So the words Jenny's mother spoke were very comforting.

Knowing that Erik was fully accepted for who he was, by someone he loved very much and her family; well that's like balm to a mother's heart. One day, Jenny said to me, "You know it's funny, but I think there's a reason that Erik and I are together now, a reason that we found each other again. I knew I loved him the very first time I saw him when we were just teenagers. There was something about him. His eyes; his eyes do the talking. Now, I see he has your eyes."

Talk about melting a mother's heart. That did it. I got to know Jenny in a whirlwind; such an intense environment and both fighting for a love we shared. That time will always be very special, just as I know that our relationship will always be very special. Jenny sent me this text six months later:

> *That day was like 9/11. You'll never forget it and wonder if it's real. You'll never forget what you were doing at the time and there is an incredible story that follows. I just wanted to thank you for being a great mother and treating me like family.*

It's not hard to treat someone like family when they act like they are. Her presence was irreplaceable. I truly believe she was the reason that Erik was still alive. He had unfinished business, the business of love and family, the business of Jenny. She's why he chose to stay. I'm sure of it.

Rehash of the Crash

April 14, 2010 at approximately 11 o'clock in the morning, Erik left class at Cape Fear Community College on his motorcycle. Nick, Erik's younger half-brother, had plans to celebrate his 14th birthday that day. Erik had plans to travel to Florida with his girlfriend Jenny, later that afternoon. There were a lot of things planned for that day, just not the event that was about to take place. Riding his motorcycle, Erik rounded the final curve of River Road, only a mile from where he lived with his father. He didn't make it through the curve. Traveling at high speed, at least 80 mph, he lost control. His body slammed against a tree, back first, with his book bag acting as yet another blunt instrument to the impact of his spine.

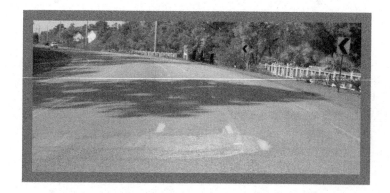

Scene of accident at River Road in Wilmington, NC
Erik's body slammed into a tree, seventy-five yards ahead

A woman traveling the opposite direction, who met Erik at the apex of the curve, was the only eyewitness. When I called her to get more information, she said it was the most horrible thing she'd ever seen. As she approached Erik coming around the bend, she saw his bike start to wobble and then watched him crash in her rear view mirror. She continued to drive and was so upset that she called her daughter. Her daughter called 911. The woman decided to turn around and go back to the scene of the accident where she prayed with the others that had gathered.

I spoke with her twice via phone and asked her to visit us, to help us understand the accident and the resulting injuries. Each time she said she would, but each time she never showed. The condition of the bike didn't reveal the violence or details of the crash. Other than Erik's body, this woman was the only thing that could tell that story. Even Erik's memory would fail him, only remembering that day to the point when he left school.

Since Erik's riding skills were excellent and he always wore full gear, Ron was on the war path and adamant to find a reason for the crash. He was not satisfied with the report from the police stating the accident was simply due to speeding. He believed that Erik was riding faster than the speed limit, but he knew Erik's high level of riding skill and his gut said that speed wasn't the single factor responsible for the accident. On his way to the hospital Thursday morning, the day after the accident, he noticed a barely visible substance spilled across the road just before the crash site, but he didn't think anything of it. Friday morning, Ron blew into the hospital with a vengeance, his eyes fiery and feverish, like a wild animal that just completed a successful hunt. "That tree took my son out, so I took that tree out!" With vengeful anger that only a father can know, he announced that no one would ever be hurt again by that tree.

I've seen that volatile look in his eyes before; it's chilling and uncontrollable. Ron couldn't sleep so he rose before the sun to cut down the tree that paralyzed his son and then kept a slice of it as booty, to give to Erik. It reminded me of a warrior bringing scalps from the enemy camp. He also started to piece together his own version of what happened.

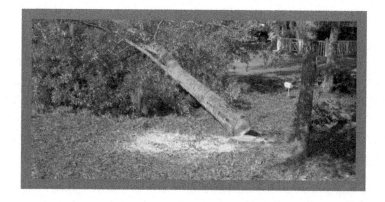

Results of Ron's rampage

The barely visible wet substance he'd seen previously across the road had dried. It was now a light color and easily visible. Ron gathered samples of the white substance and put them in the trunk of his car. He was certain it was a factor in Erik's loss of control.

I felt myself becoming nauseated. I remembered how crazed Ron was when we divorced. When he felt that he was protecting what was rightfully his, especially his son, his instincts were explosive. Nothing could stop him, trust me. Like the time when Erik was four years old and playing outside and the neighbor's two big dogs broke loose. We couldn't find Erik and felt he might be in danger. The dogs were not friendly when they were standing on our sidewalk barking.

Ron grabbed a rifle, went looking for Erik and shot one of the dogs he encountered on his quest. Not a pretty ending for the dog our relationship with the neighbors. And poor Erik had a member of that neighbor's family as his kindergarten teacher when he was five; tough way to start off the first year of school.

I was nervous and felt myself tensing up. I wanted to shut down to escape Ron's rampage but I knew I had to stay present, emotionally and physically. This was no time to zone out. Too much was at stake.

"Not now," I murmured quietly to myself. "I just can't do it." I looked at Chuck. He sensed my internalized meltdown and offered to visit the scene of the accident with Ron to take pictures and investigate the substance on the road more closely.

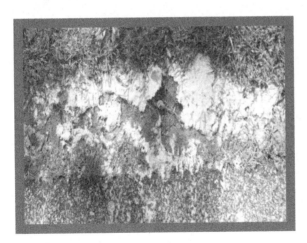

Remnants of run-off from the dried spill where Erik lost control of his motorcycle

Thank God for Chuck's intervening gesture. It gave me time to process unpleasant buried memories and it gave Ron monitored guidance through his warrior fever. At the scene, they took pictures and gathered more samples of the substance spilled across the road. It was wet and gray when he first noticed it, the same color as the pavement. By now, it was dried and white. The substance resembled paper pulp. When we added water, it became very slimy.

Police and neighbors who lived on the road did not notice it on the day of the accident. We have no proof it was there on the day of the accident. Suspicious? To us, yes. We were looking for answers – reasons, especially Ron.

Just as my motherhood instincts went into overdrive, Ron's fatherhood instincts were off the charts. I took the photos and our suspicions to the State Police barracks. The sergeant did not agree that the mystery substance could have been a factor in the crash. Was it there and not noticed because of the stopped traffic covering it or because of the shadow the trees cast on the road, which was apparent in our photographs? We'll never know. Yes, a lot of unanswered questions, but one big miracle. Erik was alive.

The unanswered
questions
lend to the
mysticism of
acceptance,

with no answers,

and what
it means to
really
move on.

Actually, the thought of what may have caused the accident made me physically ill. I knew my thyroid was already pushed to the limit so I truly had to put it all out of my mind. If I didn't, I would feel nauseated and weak. Any time it was brought up, I simply said, "It doesn't matter now. Everyone that knows Erik knows that he is a skilled rider. He has no shame. It's done and over. All that matters is that Erik is alive and with us now."

It gnawed at me, about how to move forward to find answers. I made a few legal inquiries because I wanted to pursue further investigation despite the police report. I knew if Erik survived there would be unexpected expenses that go along with a paraplegic life. But then again, we've always gotten by without much money. We're a resourceful family with loads of support. I trusted that we'd get by again, just fine, no matter what the outcome.

Nonetheless, I met with the police. That was a dead end. I realized that I had limited energy, time and resources. My top priority was Erik so I decided to focus everything I had on his recovery. I couldn't afford to waste any time or energy with attorneys, police reports, speculation or arguments.

At that point, I felt a settling in my soul. My epiphany had arrived. Unbeknownst to me, I'd actually been preparing for this mission for quite some time. I'd been doing the spiritual work of consciously developing intuitive healing gifts of Spirit for the past five years and left behind conventional methods of work to begin my Intuitive Healing Coach practice. I'd received my Coaches Certification from the International Association of Coaches and upon a suggestion from an Enneagram teacher and nun; I obtained my Reiki Master Teacher certification. Having been raised in a very rural and conservative environment, this new path was scary for me.

I'd been afraid of what others would think of me and hurt by what some had said about my *intuitive* work. Work was supposed to be about blood, sweat and tears – not intuition. That didn't follow the tradition of my German forefathers that placed hard work next to godliness.

Perhaps it took a situation as tragic as Erik's accident to shake me from my own worst enemy – me – because since the moment I got the call, I was living completely in the moment and from my heart instead of my head. It was exactly what my thyroid called for; to speak and live my truth. I couldn't care less about what anybody thought or said. I'd embraced my mission.

The parts of my spiritual work that others might not understand; the intuitive seeing, the stones, the reiki, the oils, the movements of my hands, were now the very tools that I would draw upon. I *knew* my Jesus, my Christ, my Holy Spirit, my Guides and Guardians; and all are of Divine Love, One with my God. There was no doubt, no fear, no hesitation and no time for anything except facilitating Erik's healing. That was my purpose, the most profound purpose I'd ever been called for.

Throughout this ordeal, many people asked if I would forbid Erik to ride motorcycle again. As an ex-rider myself, I've experienced the joy of riding. I may have hoped that Erik would give it up, but I would never say so. Even if I did forbid him, he wouldn't listen anyway. Erik's choices may impact me in a devastating way, yet they are still his choices, his consequences. My responsibility lies with my own choices, including how I respond to things that are devastating.

The questions about forbidding him to ride again prompted me to revisit a Facebook conversation I had with Erik and one of his friends, Bryan, just three months before the crash.

Erik's Facebook

Erik Fugunt

Posted this photo January 21, 2010 at 4:15pm

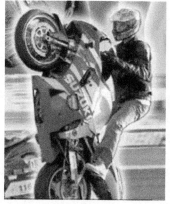

Like · Comment · Share

Jacqueline Dunkle

...just wondering Erik. Is that you in the wheelie pic? Remember the "endo" you did when I was following you at Daytona Beach for your graduation? you got my heart going ... as usual

January 21, 2010 at 6:22pm

Erik Fugunt

Yeah that was me at MIR it was a wheelie contest

January 21, 2010 at 6:45pm

Jacqueline Dunkle

very cool. I've been thinking about your antics all day - like when you used to jump the sidewalk at the Aframe with the little Honda 50 - and did you crash one time - because of the kitty cat?

January 21, 2010 at 6:50pm

Erik Fugunt

I always crash over a cat ... but yeah I remember that lol...

January 21, 2010 at 6:52pm

Bryan

how do you do it jacque? My mom would keel over if she ever witnessed me do anything like that. erik, your mom is a strong woman for putting up with your dangerous endeavors.
January 21, 2010 at 7:04pm

Jacqueline Dunkle

Witnessing someone completely "present within their Essence" is like witnessing God in the flesh. I feel a sense of awe not fear when I see my beloved son in his "zone". My fear had to be surrendered to the grace of faith that assures me death cannot ever separate our souls or our love.
January 21, 2010 at 7:17pm

Erik Fugunt

That's why I love my mom! She gets it!
January 21, 2010 at 7:19pm

Bryan

*closes eyes, breathes deep, spine tingles * YESS!!
January 21, 2010 at 7:24pm

Erik Fugunt

haha, love ya bryan!
January 21, 2010 at 7:35pm

I got it alright. And I was getting it now, like never before. I didn't like it, but I got. And Bryan's spine was tingling, but Erik's spine wasn't feeling anything at all – it couldn't.

Erik's choices were just that, his choices. Of course he never dreamed he would be paralyzed by consequence of choice. He thought the consequence would be death. We all did. Somehow we'd all been able to accept that. But how do we accept paralysis? How do we accept the fact that he won't be able to walk, urinate, defecate and inseminate? Oh man, this was gonna be a stretch. I knew, or hoped, that we could adjust but I also knew it was going to be the hardest adjustment any of us had ever experienced, especially Erik, of course. So I got it. And even though I did not want my son to experience the hardships of paralysis, I did not want him to die. So I prayed for him to live. Then I prayed for grace to accept the outcome; death or life and paralysis.

The Awakening

Friday morning, day three, was the first time I was finally alone in a private place and felt safe enough to break down, to surrender. I was in the shower of the Wilmington Hospitality House ladies bathroom. I began sobbing in despair and disbelief, hoping the hot water that trickled over my body would somehow warm the cold dark place that I was walking through; the place that I came to know as the Valley of the Shadow of Death. I bawled and bawled and gasped for air, again and again, praying the 23rd Psalm and crying out to God for help, "Please help me. Please, please help my son. Please help him. Please help us."

As I continued to sob, I began to sing something from out of the blue, "And I will raise him up. And I will raise him up. And I will raise him up on the right day." Of course, Christ lives out of the blue. I knew where the song had come from. The original song sings, "I will raise him up on the LAST day", but I kept singing "I will raise him up on the RIGHT day." I looked it up on YouTube when I began to write this chapter. It's a song by Suzanne Toolan entitled *I am the Bread of Life*. I hadn't heard that song for about thirty years, but I heard it like bells ringing in my head that morning. And all I could do was sing it over and over, sputtering the words and tune from my lips that were covered in hot water and snot, from the shower and from my tears. I was a mess, humbled and naked before my God. And God came to me in song, helping me surrender all and giving me an affirmation to claim.

During that musical shower mess, I was gently interrupted by a woman's voice, "Are you okay, honey?" I caught my breath immediately. I was busted; caught bawling and moaning like a little baby. "Yes," I sheepishly echoed from behind the shower curtain. You know how a baby tries to catch their breath in between sobs? Well that was me. "I'm okay. (gasp) My son (gasp, gasp) was in a motorcycle accident. (gasp) I'll be okay."

"Alright," she replied. "If there's anything I can do to help, just let me know." She didn't know it but she'd already done what I needed. I thought the shower curtain would protect me from the outside world and from looking vulnerable. Her kind words gently awakened me from my pride; they reminded me that I would not get through this alone. I wanted to be strong but strength does not come from being alone and independent. It comes from surrendering and accepting help. I would be needing help from many people to navigate through this Dark Valley.

We counted the hours and then the days. Saturday, day four, my brother Tim and his wife Patty flew in from Dallas. We all prayed reverently, constantly touching Erik with hands of love. I softly sang favorite hymns and childhood songs to him around the clock. Friends of Ron's also joined us and surrounded Erik in prayer. I swear I couldn't keep my hands from touching his precious body. I used my stones and offered reiki via my Christian faith, asking the Holy Spirit to use my body as a clear vessel to share the healing Light and Love of Christ with Erik, according to his highest purpose at this time. You know, that's pretty hard to say and very hard to pray because my ego had its own idea of what was best for Erik, *what I wanted*. So my prayers and healing hands practice were beneficial for me as well. They helped me surrender to God, whatever the outcome.

At 8:30 a.m. on Sunday morning, day five, Chuck and I stepped into Erik's ICU room. I did the first thing I always did. I leaned to kiss him and studied every detail of his face. Having gone into my zone, I didn't notice anything different until Ron said, "Jacq, don't you notice anything?" He was grinning. He hadn't left Erik's side all night. It felt good to know that he was vigilantly watching over Erik when I tried to rest.

"What?" I stood up and stepped back with a quizzical look on my face, "What?" I asked again.

"Didn't you notice? He's not shaking! They changed him from the infant respirator, the oscillator, to the adult respirator." Ron's grin was priceless. It worked. Erik's left lung, which had fallen out of his chest in pieces just a few days ago, had somehow healed enough to hold air with an adult respirator. "Oh my God, you've got to be kidding me!" My face lit up like a Christmas tree. Sure enough, his body was no longer shaking like a robot. The air compressor puffing noise from the oscillator was silent. Dear God, he made it over one more hurdle. I couldn't believe it. I looked around the room to make sure I was in the right place.

I asked Louise when she changed respirators. "About 8 o'clock this morning." she replied with a big smile. It was the exact time that friends of mine were holding a Native American healing ceremony for Erik back in Pennsylvania. How's that for serendipity? Since the doctors didn't expect him to survive the whole ordeal, it was obvious that Erik was doing better than they anticipated. They were shocked and amazed with his rapid progress, so they decided to go for the switch in respirators sooner than planned. Erik's lungs cooperated completely. The hurdles that lie ahead were numerous, but we still had hope. Each day was a balancing act of hope versus hurdles, benefits versus risks, life versus death.

Jenny was lamenting that afternoon. She needed to make the three hour drive home to Mebane, back to her job, classes and finals. Her heart was sickened. She didn't want to leave Erik. "What if he wakes up and I'm not here? I don't want him to think that I left him." She was torn between her heart and her logistical life. I promised her that I would tell him how she stayed around the clock to be with him. And how she told me in the waiting room that she knew she loved him the very first time she saw him ten years ago, when they were just teenagers. She decided to stay and drive back later that night.

Thank goodness, or she would have missed the awakening. I stepped outside at around 6 p.m. to get a breath of fresh air when my brother Tim, came to find me. "They're looking for you. They're going to try and wake him up." My eyes just about popped out of my head.

They had placed Erik on drugs to intentionally paralyze his entire body in order to keep him still and allow his damaged lung time to heal. They were going to lift the intentional paralysis and sedation to see if Erik would respond to voice commands. Initial scans did not reveal any brain damage but since his brain had been without oxygen for an extended period of time during the initial trauma, brain damage could not be ruled out.

I literally sprinted down the hallway to the ICU where I stood frozen with bated breath. There was a part of me that didn't want this to happen. I was able to see and kiss my son's face. I was able to be near him. I was able to be present with him. I was able to hope. Let's not change that. Let's not see if he can respond. Maybe he can't. Maybe he does have brain damage from the horrendous impact or from lack of oxygen. Maybe we should just let well enough alone. Honestly, I can't explain the terror of that moment.

Holding his left hand, Louise, our ICU sunshine, said with a loud voice, "Erik, squeeze my hand." I held my breath and waited. Nothing. "Erik," she spoke again, even louder and with more intensity. "Erik, if you can hear me, please, squeeze my hand." Still nothing. She paused. Everyone in the room was gathered around, pulling for him, rooting for him; the body language and thoughts whispering, "Come on Erik. You can do it. Come on."

Then Louise firmly commanded him, "Erik, honey, squeeze my hand."

Still breathless, we all waited and watched.

Oh my God! His fingers moved! He's trying to squeeze! My heart exploded with joy. My eyes exploded with tears. He did it! He tried to squeeze her hand! His brain is working! He's able to respond! I turned to hug Jenny and lifted her right off the ground. My voice was a jubilant whisper, "He did it! He did it!" The room was filled with a whispering celebration suitable for intensive care surroundings. Remember how Erik had told the inquiring visitor from Ireland in the restaurant three weeks ago that his head was worth protecting? Things that make you go, "Hmm…" We found out later that the hand she was squeezing and he tried to move, was broken as well; an oversight because of all the other life threatening injuries.

 Jenny and me,

celebrating in the ICU waiting room, after Erik responds

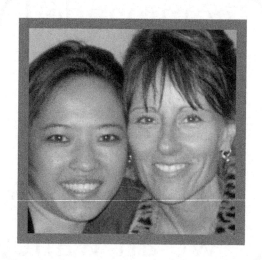

I knew that Erik could hear us talking to him over the past four days. The monitors would reveal an increase in his heart rate when certain people would say things to him. And once when I was singing to him, I swear a tear welled up and seeped from his closed eyes. I knew he could hear us at some level. But now, knowing that he was able to acknowledge our voices and respond, oh dear Lord, thank you, thank you. That was the warmest I ever was in the ICU. It was always freezing in there, so I was always bundled up in hoodies, sweaters and scarves. But jumping up and down in celebration, like a delighted child on Christmas morning helped warm me up and Erik's response warmed me even deeper. Oddly enough, though, I still had an unsettling feeling, the same one I'd get when he was a sleeping baby and I was afraid he'd awaken. "Oh dear," I thought. "Please don't wake him up yet. All hell breaks loose when he's awake. I'd like to enjoy this blissful moment."

Now the plan would be to back off on the meds, allow Erik to drift in and out of consciousness and continue to look for responses to commands and voices. That was enough for tonight. He'd passed the first test of response. Maybe the helmet worked.

That night, Jenny drove back to Mebane, Chuck and I stayed at the Hospitality House with my brother and sister-in-law and Ron stayed with Erik. Even though I wanted to be the one to stay with Erik, I needed food and rest. Watching Ron caress Erik's face reminded me that I had loved that man. He'd lean over the bed and say "I love you, Erik. You're my best buddy." He was crazy Ron, yes. But he loved his son, dearly.

Monday, day six, brought a changing of the guard. Lori, my right hand friend, arrived from Pittsburgh with more supplies since this was obviously going to be a long term tour of duty. Before she made the drive down, we talked via cell phone while she was at my house packing more clothes for me. At the time, Erik was still on the oscillator and we had no idea how he was going to progress. I remember asking her if I should have dress clothes, in case there was a funeral. "No," she quickly dictated the plan. "We'll get dress clothes there, if we have to." She unselfishly and admirably rose to the occasion amidst the grief that still shrouded her from the loss of her son in an accident just 11 months earlier.

As fate would have it, when Lori arrived Chuck had to leave. His employer called and wanted him in Harrisburg until further notice. It seemed like such heartless, horrible timing but truthfully, it worked out for the best. Aside from Chuck having to live in a hotel hundreds of miles away and not being able to see us, it was okay. I knew that my immediate orders were signed, sealed and delivered. I would not be leaving Wilmington until Erik was well or gone, or both. Either way, my life would be consumed with Erik's care, 24/7 just as it was destined to be, for his and my healing. The nursing staff kept reminding me to get my rest, that I'd need it down the road.

I knew they were right but I also knew my nature. I tend to be a taskmaster, workaholic, over achiever, whatever you want to call it. If I had those characteristics to begin with, you can imagine what a catalyst this situation was. I was definitely in overdrive. It's kind of crazy when I think about it now; how even though I had my moments of breakdown, for the most part I was like a machine, just doing what I thought needed to be done.

At any rate, before Chuck left that day he stood at Erik's bedside rallying him with these words, "I love you Erik. You can do this. And remember; pain heals, chicks dig scars and glory is forever." With a sense of helplessness, Chuck got into the car with my brother who took him to the airport. There seemed to be a lesson in all this for Chuck too. His lesson was wrapped up in his deep desire to help others at any cost, to take care of them and make things better. But there are just some things you can't make better; things that make or break us. And we had a whopper of one of those things in our face, just waiting to define us. Chuck was so sweet and patient with me. Over the next three months, I had minimal contact with him; one, maybe two brief phone calls a day. When we did speak on the phone, we were often interrupted by the task at hand. When our conversation wasn't cut short by an interruption, my attention span was so short or I was so exhausted that I didn't even feel like talking.

His support and understanding, even from a distance was wonderful. He kept a daily journal of each day's happenings and distributed it via email. I referenced that journal as I wrote this book, to help me remember. So in his own way, he helped more than he could ever imagine.

My brother Tim and his wife Patty, who'd flown in from Dallas, were preparing to return home as well. They'd stood by Erik's bedside praying over him, gently telling him they loved him. They encouraged him, "You can do this. Keep fighting Erik. And believe."

When they said goodbye, Erik didn't speak, nor was he completely conscious, but he unexpectedly and triumphantly raised his right arm high, as if to say goodbye or show his fighting spirit. We didn't know which. What we did know was that this battle wasn't over. Our Erik Wolfgang was the underdog, but he was gaining ground.

Over the next few days, as Erik became more aware, he began to attempt communication. He was responding to commands, as much as his broken body would allow. I think it was Monday, day six, the first time he tried to speak to me. We were alone. He opened his eyes and saw me in the room. He began to cry. It was horrible. Tears were streaming down the sides of his face past the feeding tube that was taped to his cheek. He couldn't talk so he began to mouth words, "I'm so sorry. I screwed up. I'm so sorry. I love you." I assured him that he didn't screw up. That it was just an accident, that I loved him. And that all he needed to do was rest and get stronger. I quietly told him the story of Doctor Mindy and the trauma team; how they saved his life. He cried and mouthed the words, "I'm so sorry, Mama. I'm so sorry. I love you." He was so hopped up on drugs, I wasn't sure if he'd be able to remember the story about Doctor Mindy. So on Tuesday morning, day seven, when she stopped to check on him, when Erik opened his eyes, I said, "Erik, this is Doctor Mindy. She is the one I've been telling you about."

"Hi Erik," she greeted him with a kind but strictly professional demeanor. Erik began to slowly lift his right arm toward where she was standing at his bedside, so she stepped closer. He reached up and gently cradled her face in his hand. I could see him trying to talk past the tracheotomy and respirator. So I intently watched his lips. With his hand still tenderly holding Doctor Mindy's face, his lips struggled but slowly and successfully made the outline of these words, "Thank... you...for....saving...my...life."

I almost died myself. If I never live to see another sun set, I'll swear I'll have already witnessed the most endearing and humbling connection that a human can experience. I repeated his words out loud for him, to validate what I had just witnessed. "Thank you for saving my life." He slowly nodded yes. Doctor Mindy's professional face melted like ice cubes in sunshine. It was a sight to behold. Erik had not only won a physical victory in the trauma bay, he'd won her heart as well. She explained that a lot of people were responsible for his being here, not claiming any glory for herself. Then Erik dozed off. It was such an intimate tender moment; our hearts had been touched in the most profound way. He thanked her for saving his life, but he didn't know about the paralysis yet. I hoped he'd still be thankful when he did.

The Healing Room

For two days between full coma and full consciousness, Erik was being weaned from the same drug that killed Michael Jackson – Propofol. We called it the Michael Jackson Magic Sleeping Drug. He would drift in and out a lot. He would open his eyes and see me and start to cry. Due to the tracheotomy and respirator, communication was next to impossible. We gave him a paper and pencil but he was so banged and drugged up, he couldn't write legibly enough for us to read; well truthfully, even when he's not banged up it's tough to read his chicken scratch. He quickly became disgusted and frustrated and threw the pencil; though he only had the ability to throw it as far as his own lap. The look in his eyes said it all. Jenny was right. His eyes did talk and what they said broke my heart. There was nothing I could do to help him, but just be there.

His inability to communicate with paper and pencil fueled the fire for his attempts to speak verbally. He mouthed words and tried his best to talk past the tracheotomy and respirator. I could understand most of his mouthing but it made the message even more pathetic as he struggled to communicate. He mouthed things to me that he would never say if he were in his right, non-drugged mind. He was so humble and so darn sweet, not his ordinary ornery self at all. "I'm so sorry. I'm so sorry. I screwed up." His mouth made the shapes of the words.

Again, I tenderly explained to him that he didn't screw up. That it was just an accident and all of us have accidents. There was no need for him to be sorry. All he had to do was rest, get stronger and use his energy to heal. Then he shifted his eyes to look around the room. He saw all the ICU contraptions and panicked.

He emphatically mouthed, "I can't pay for all this. We don't have enough money to pay for this!" His eyes grew huge as he continued to lip synch his words. I told him not to worry. That it was all taken care of and he just needed to rest and get stronger. His eyes didn't let up. He must have thought we bartered our organs to pay for the hospital services because he mouthed "What did you do? How did you take care of it? You don't have enough money."

I explained that I wasn't paying for it. I didn't have to do anything but help his dad with some paperwork. He was eligible for Medicaid. They would pay for his care. Kind of funny, but some of my hardworking family said they were glad to see someone they loved make use of their tax dollars after so many years of contributing to the fund. His eyes finally relaxed. But he continued to mouth.

"I'm so sorry. I love you, Mom. But, how are we going to do this?"

I looked him dead straight in the eyes, and said with full resolve,

"Erik, we can do this. Just believe."

He mouthed back emphatically, "I believe. But how? How are we going to do this?"

I replied truthfully, with conviction and a piercing look from my eyes to his, "*With strength, determination and love; and we've got lots of that.*" Then he drifted off, his sad eyes closed and my sad heart ached. But I meant every word.

I observed his behavior closely those few days. I was able to bask in a part of my son's essence that I'd forgotten about. During that short period of time, he didn't cry or expose his vulnerability to anyone but me. He was a tough guy with everyone else. I had his sweetness all to myself and if only for a few days, it was enough to last a lifetime. His tenderness and humility were palpable.

I'd been given an incredible gift, the gift of revisiting a tender time of just "being" with my son, a time of soft and quiet nurturing, a time that was overshadowed in his childhood by the power and fun of Dad and the heaviness of responsibility. I allowed those healing moments to seat themselves deeply in my heart. The next time he drove me crazy, I'd remember the soothing sweetness of his being that lingers just beneath the surface.

Apparently, Erik wouldn't remember any of it because on Wednesday morning, day eight, he asked his dad if I had been contacted. "Erik, she's been here for a week now, since the night of the accident! Don't you remember? You're on some good drugs. She just went to get a shower. She'll be back." When I returned from my shower, Ron told me he didn't remember my being there. I kissed him all over again and told him how much I loved him and that he was going to be alright. We told him how wonderful Jenny had been and that she stayed by his side for five days but had to drive back to Mebane for school and work. We assured him that she'd be returning to see him as soon as she could and she wanted him to know that she didn't leave him. His eyes would fill with tears. I'm not sure he believed us. Erik was beginning to get a sense of his surroundings, his body and the severity of his accident. He was feeling the pain of his physical injuries but was heartsick about Jenny and the future of their relationship as well.

He was becoming much more cognizant now. But it was hard to communicate. Success in that area depended on Erik's degree of lucidness and our ability to lip read, which became very frustrating for all. It took a long time for us to figure out that he wanted his father on one side and me on the other.

Then he grabbed each of our arms to help him reposition himself in the bed. The drugs obviously helped dull the pain of movement that he would have normally felt from his injuries. "We make a good team," he mouthed. It was reminiscent of a time when we were a team and not living the lives of a divorced family. All for one, one for all, together with all the attention placed on the well-being of our only child.

That night, we started into a new routine. Typically, Ron would sleep in a chair in Erik's room and I would go to the Hospitality House about 10:45 p.m. because of an 11:00 p.m. curfew. That night, as we began those proceedings, Erik began to fuss and complain about his stomach. He mouthed that he couldn't breathe. His father and I tried to convince him that he was breathing, that the respirator would ensure it, even if he didn't feel like he was. He was very anxious and I was too.

I silently wondered if his lung was collapsing. Then I began to massage his stomach and noticed how distended it was. He looked pregnant, with a big old tummy sticking up from his broken body. The massaging seemed to help, if not physically, at least emotionally, so I continued.

"Dad," Erik mouthed. "You go home and get some sleep. Mom, can you stay with me?"

Could I stay with him? Are you kidding? He's coherent and he wants me to stay with him? Halleluiah! My day of being Mom had come!

My baby wants me! Obviously, I tried to be cool about it when I said, "Of course, honey. As long as it takes, I'll stay with you. I'm not going anywhere." So his dad reluctantly left by Erik's direct request.

In retrospect, this was an interesting turn of events. Seventeen years ago, Erik didn't want anything to do with me. He was hurt then and felt he was abandoned by me. He kept me at bay for many years. I, on the other hand, craved to be his mother. I missed so much of his life, especially when he and Ron moved from Pennsylvania to North Carolina. But I accepted the pain as penance for my decision to get a divorce. Perhaps each of us needed to find the missing piece of those years apart. Perhaps this change of events, my staying with Erik instead of Ron, was that missing piece; a chance to be together, rebuild trust, nurture love. None of this was a consideration at the time, for any of us. It just seems strange how the events unfolded and how choices that were made corresponded with past crossroads.

It was time for his dad to go home. Ron had promised that he would not leave Erik's side until he woke up. He'd kept that promise and only went home for an occasional shower or short nap. It was time for him to resume some type of normal work schedule. He had a wife and family at home that counted on him for their care as well. I, on the other hand, had nothing but time; no work that couldn't be postponed, no other children, nothing. It was all about my son's life now. I was fortunate to be in a position that allowed me to stay and my heart goes out to those that don't have that option. I wondered if it was even an option. I would have given up anything – job, house, and spouse – to stay with my child. Fortunately, my relationship with Chuck was strong and based on values that would support my decision to stay with Erik as long as it took.

So there I was in the wee hours of the night, massaging Erik's distended tummy, when *he* figured out what was causing his labored breath. Keep in mind that he was hooked up to the respirator so he communicated by mouthing. I was able to interpret most of his words by now, but it was still like playing charades a lot of the time. "I can't breathe," he mouthed. He reached to touch his stomach where he still had feeling. "Like I'm too full. Are they feeding me?"

"Yes, through that tube in your nose." I answered him. He reached to touch his nose and felt the small tube. I could see the wheels turning in his head. I knew that look.

"Make them stop." he demanded via mouthing. "Make them stop. I can't breathe."

I called for the nurse and explained the situation to her. Of course she couldn't disobey doctor's orders. She tried to convince Erik that she couldn't stop feeding him. And the battle began.

"You have to stop feeding me," he pleaded with a demanding look. "I can't breathe. Look at my stomach! It's huge. You're over feeding me. I can't breathe."

The respirator ensured that Erik would continue to breath but his body clearly told him that his breathing was being impaired. His distended stomach was putting too much pressure on his lungs. He had the same sensation that you would have after you've eaten too much on Thanksgiving Day, only worse because his lungs were compromised. I attempted to reason with the nurse. "Can't you just stop for a while? Give him a break?"

The nurse came right back at us with her ammunition of hierarchy. "No, I really can't stop it. It's what the doctor ordered. And I have to follow the order."

Erik looked around at all the gadgets and bags hanging at his bedside. He saw the bag of food and his eyes followed the tube from the bag to his nose where he put his hand on it and lip-synched, "How does it work? Are you pumping it into me?"

"Yes," the nurse replied.

"Then reverse the pump and suck some out. You have to. I can't breathe." I had to translate his words for the nurse. Erik held the feeding tube tightly now. She started to refuse the request again so I began to plead his case. I nearly demanded that she suck some of the bag food out of his stomach, because I knew he would rip that feeding tube out of his nose if she didn't. His talking eyes and firm grip on the feeding tube confirmed my words. I convinced her that we can always put more back in if we need to. I wasn't backing down.

She finally agreed to suck it back out. Thank God! With each measurable amount she removed, Erik felt relief and encouraged her to keep going. She eventually removed enough to satisfy him and said she would speak to the doctor about changing the amount of food that was being administered.

When the nurse left the room Erik took my hand and mouthed, "You can't leave me alone, Mom. Please stay with me. I don't trust them. They won't listen to me."

Even though there were no sounds with those words coming from his lips, I heard him, loud and clear. He was scared. He knew that some heroic feats had been done to save his life, but he also knew his own body. At that point, I realized that not only was I Erik's mother, I was also his patient advocate and Intuitive Healing Coach. And boy was I ready for the job.

"I'm not going anywhere Erik. I'll be right here with you as long as it takes. I promise." I wholeheartedly believed in Erik and his ability to sense what was happening in his body. It coincided completely with my work as an Intuitive Healing Coach.

And I wondered if perhaps I had been chosen for this exact task. Because as crazy as it sounds, these next two photos were taken during an annual visit to Baja Mexico, at a town named Todos Santos – meaning *All Saints*. It was February of 2010, just weeks before Erik's accident. I noticed a carving of Christ's face in a tree stump at the Emporium next to Hotel California.

It was unbelievably beautiful. And it was unbelievably growing new life; a cut off piece of tree stump was able to provide enough substance to grow a bright green leafy twig! New life from death.

I was completely entranced with it and could hardly tear myself away from it. Chuck took pictures as I kneeled reverently in front of the stump. I shared the photos with a Shaman during my search for natural treatment of my hyperthyroid. She saw symbolisms etched in the nuances of the trunk; a wolf, a reiki symbol and most fascinating – a Medicine Woman standing over a sick man wrapped in a blanket.

She felt that the stump and the symbols held very specific messages for me. Wow. And look at me now; standing over my son wrapped in blankets; my son whom I named Erik *Wolf*gang; holding tight to my faith in Christ and sharing reiki. And the Shaman saw it all, in that stump. Who says there's no modern day prophecy?

The Shaman saw these and many more symbols in that stump, just weeks before the accident. It's taken some time for me to see them clearly, but now they appear distinctly to my eyes. I know that sometimes we see what we want to see, or can't see what we don't want to see; that we all "see" with different eyes, different hearts.

The stump with symbols circled on the side of Christ's face

Top circle
the wolf

2nd circle
the reiki symbol

3ᵣ circle
the medicine woman
standing above
blanketed man

Bottom circle
the man wrapped
in blankets
head tilted down in
right side of circle

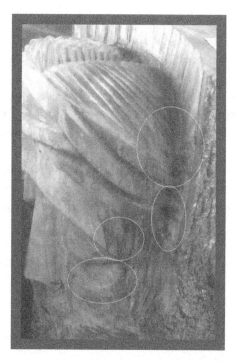

So believe what you will, but I believe there was a message etched out for me in that beautiful stump. I felt the grace of God shine into me when I knelt at the Face of Christ that day. And now that grace would carry me though this difficult healing journey with my son. It was my divine purpose.

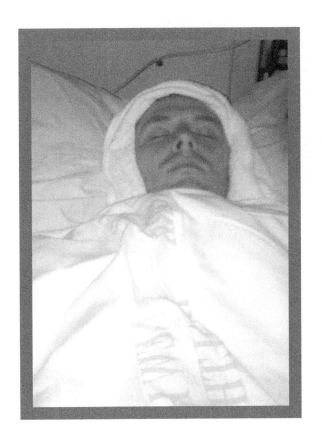

My son wrapped in a blankets,

just like the man in the stump

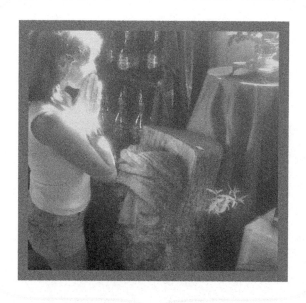

Me, kneeling at the Face of Christ
carved into the tree stump

I have no logical explanation for how my own compromised health
and strength were holding up. Support frequently arrived at the
Hospitality House from friends and family; in the form of cards, care
packages and even monetary gifts. My hyperthyroid symptoms were
less severe than they had been when I left Pennsylvania. I was still
experiencing fatigue and throat discomfort, but I was managing.
And I told nobody. A few weeks prior, my thyroid's THS level was
.01. Normal range is .5 to 4.5 so I was next to nil. I stayed the course
with natural modalities and continued taking a thyroid supplement,
vitamin D3, a multivitamin and B12 drops. I also drank hot water
every morning laced with a few drops of motherwort to relieve
heart palpitations. I used Nyquil occasionally, to induce short
afternoon naps. And I took a few hours for myself, away from the
hospital to receive massage and acupuncture.

When I asked a nurse if I could bring the massage therapist into the hospital for Erik, I was shocked and excited to learn that this little hospital in Wilmington, New Hanover Regional Medical Center, had a Healing Arts Department! All we had to do was request massage therapy and they would provide it for him. Who knew? So Erik received massage therapy from Marilyn, the hospital's therapist, while in ICU and throughout his entire hospital stay. They also provided healing touch therapy and constant gentle healing music in his room.

We literally turned Erik's ICU room into a healing room. My medicine woman roots took hold of that space. Every card, every email, every little thing of love and support that could be, was taped to the walls and doorway of that room until there was practically no wall space left.

There were balloons, plants, flowers, baseball caps and posters that came from his college classmates, family and friends. Placed throughout the room and taped to his bed were crystals. One came from his English professor, a very special woman, Ms. Ach who visited Erik faithfully. I put Jenny's picture in a frame that was embossed with the word "LOVE" and positioned it so that Erik could see it when he opened his eyes. Amulets and gifts from healers that were gathered from sacred places were sent to us. I hung the Japanese symbol of "Miracle" in his room.

I always kept my stones and Grandma's bell in my purse so they were with me when I arrived in Wilmington. My Grandmother Schrecengost had a string of bells hanging from her door. When she crossed over, I was able to keep the old bells. I put them on my door to keep her love and spirit close. The string that held them together was so old and frayed that one of the bells fell off. So I decided to use it as a tool for my energy work. What better energy to be present at all times than Grandma Schrec's love?

She'd lost two sons to tragic accidents, so she was more than seasoned with despair and loss, yet managed to live a long life. With Erik, I'd sometimes ring it to summon her love and I'd sometimes just hold it or place it on his body.

I must say, it wasn't the norm compared to the other ICU rooms. But the staff was respectful and even allowed privacy for other natural treatments that I brought in for Erik. I found a local healer and asked her to visit Erik. She would tap tuning forks and hold them on different acupressure points of Erik's body and around his energy field. He could feel the vibration throughout his body and it would relax him.

The nurses would enter his room and say, "Oh, it smells so good in this room. I wish I could hang out here for a while." Erik didn't necessarily agree with them. He loved the massage work, healing touch and the tuning forks, but he complained that the essential oils were stinky. The healer used oils to prevent blood clots, boost his immune system and promote relaxation. His body generated an overwhelming intense heat from some of the oils, so by his orders, we didn't use many. Upon recommendation of the healer, I continued to use Helichrysum, an essential oil used for its various healing properties.

One thing's for sure, ICU Room 8 was like no other in the unit. It was figuratively and literally filled with natural healing powers of love; not just mine or those that came in and out of that room; love was pouring into that room from across the map. Family and friends were sending gobs of it in the form of prayers, cards, texts and phone messages. A dear friend from my childhood, Kelly, held me up via the phone lines. She would call and leave a message in the form of a prayer. I'd replay it again and again, listening to her dear voice and her prayers, allowing myself to be with her in Spirit. I did the same with my Pastor Sam's prayer message.

By now, Erik was acknowledging all voice commands and trying his best to respond. But I knew that we weren't *out of the woods* yet. Doctor Mindy confirmed that. The medical staff would say, "He's one sick young man." I'd think to myself, "What do they mean 'sick'? He's injured, not sick." I guess it's a matter of semantics. And I was forgetting that the injuries were breeding grounds for sickness.

During prayer and reiki, I would place one stone in particular on his forehead, between his toes, or on his chest by the damaged lung. The lung was of major concern and no surgery would be done on his spine until his fever was diminished. Because of the unsterile environment and radical fashion in which they had to act in order to save his life, an infection in his lungs was inevitable and pneumonia was a certainty; not a good scenario anytime, let alone for a shredded lung that had been stitched up. There was even brief consideration of removing that lung, but it never came to that. I can remember one of Erik's friends watching me as I did energy work on his lungs, moving my hands over that area and lifting the infection from his body. He looked at me with skeptical but inquisitive eyes and asked, "Will that help?"

I tilted my head pensively and replied, "It won't hurt." I'd also visualize myself as part of his body at a cellular level, then enter the lungs and visualize them as healthy and pink. I would tell Erik to repeat these words, "I am healing. My lungs are pink and healthy. I am healing. My lungs are pink and healthy."

Erik continued to battle the fever for over a week and was treated with antibiotics. Another CAT scan was done to ensure there was no other reason for the fever or a different origin of infection. Nothing showed. He fought the infection and pneumonia. And just like he'd been doing all along, Erik prevailed. His fight for life continued.

That Moment

I was almost frozen, thinking about *that moment*; that God-awful ugly moment that we had to tell Erik about his legs not working, let alone the loss of body functions from his waist down. My dread was bypassed by actions beyond my control. As fate would have it, I'd gone to the Hospitality House to shower when on Thursday, eight days after the accident, a neurosurgeon entered the room to prepare Erik for a pending surgery that would stabilize his spine and simply told Erik that he was paralyzed. Just like that. I was furious. I wanted to mitigate the language that was used because I don't believe anyone but God has the final word of Erik's ability to walk again. That would be between him and God. I couldn't even say the word - *paralyzed*. I referred to his condition as, "Not able to use his legs". Perhaps because of my perspective, it was intentional that I wasn't there when they told him. I may have choked somebody. When I went to take a shower, I'd asked my friend Lori to sit with Erik to help suction his mouth and throat. So she and Erik's father were there for that horrible moment - when the neurosurgeon just walked in and told Erik that he was paralyzed from the waist down and wouldn't walk again.

There's nothing quite like the cold hard truth to bring you back to reality from the land of sweetness and humility. It wasn't a hard jump for Erik. He's a realist by nature, not one to pussyfoot around. He sees things as black or white. He wanted a second opinion, still making his requests via mouthing words and not speaking. The neurosurgeon agreed to a second opinion but assured Erik that there was no chance of him ever walking again. The second neurosurgeon's opinion later concurred.

Erik made innuendos after the neurosurgeon left the room, about everyone being better off if he were dead; precisely what I was afraid of. Lori was quick to lay into him about being dead and spoke with first-hand experience since not even a year had passed since her son's death.

"Don't *ever* say that again, Erik. No parent should bury a child, ever. It's going to be hard but you're gonna do fine Erik. You're alive for a reason. And no one would ever be better off with you being dead." Her commanding voice was filled with a grieving mother's passion and tears filled her eyes. Lori was as much of a realist as Erik, maybe even more. God, I'm glad she was there in place of me.

His father echoed Lori's message and tears. "Erik, don't *ever* think that I would be better off without you. I would be way worse off if you were dead. I'm best off, because you are still alive and here with me. I'd be no good without you. I don't know what I'd do without you. You're my best friend ever, my best buddy." Erik knew that his father spoke the absolute truth. But we all knew, and no one knew better than Erik, that it was going to be one hell of a tough haul.

I had just finished showering when Lori called me and filled me in on the scene. I was sick to my stomach. By the time I'd made it back to the ICU room, their tears had been shed and dried. The shock had set in. Erik's sweetness and humility had been replaced by a distant look of angry devastation.

I felt so helpless, so useless, so horribly sad, but also relieved because the white elephant topic of paralysis was exposed. I was more afraid of what Erik might do to himself, or what he might talk his friends into doing to him, than I was of his actual paralysis.

I could figure out the logistics of a paraplegic life and do something with it, but I couldn't control what happened between Erik and his friends. I learned that lesson many years ago. It frightened me; a fear in need of healing. What better arena to bring that fear to light? Or should I say *The Light*? I had to live it now. Feel it. Become it. Surrender it.

When I entered his room, I could barely say anything. I certainly didn't say the word – *paralyzed*. I looked into his eyes and smiled and told him I loved him. For the next week, fear touched every cell of my body. I still saw my son as complete and perfect, even though motionless in a hospital bed, still whole and perfect. And I told him so. He acknowledged my perception of the situation but conveyed that my perception wasn't his reality.

I'm guessing that my son saw and felt himself in a very different way, incomplete and imperfect, certainly nothing like the young man he was just a week ago. That was reality and that was the first of the worst days ahead. The emotional pain was overbearing. It's one thing to see and know that your child is in an ICU bed, teetering between life and paralysis or death. That emotional pain is your own.

It's quite another thing to witness your child *know* that not only is he teetering between life and death but that the option of life will leave him without the use of his lower body. Your child's pain compounds with yours and exponentially increases your own emotional pain; a weighted sadness of no words and immeasurable proportion.

One evening while
I was alone with Erik
in his ICU room,

he mouthed to me
with tear-glossed
eyes,

"Mom, will you
hold me?
I forget what it
feels like to
be held."

I too, had forgotten what it felt like to hold him. Of course, I hugged him as often as I could, but I'm talking about *holding* him. I was being given the opportunity to *hold* him again; like a mother tenderly holds her baby to keep it safe. I got as close as I could to him and held him tenderly and securely as I kissed his forehead. "It's gonna be okay, Erik. I love you. It's gonna be okay." That's a moment I will treasure as long as my heart still beats.

Even though I'd been touching Erik delicately since his first day in ICU, I hadn't wrapped my arms around his entire body and held him completely, since...well, since he was a little boy. He needed the healing power of love that is delivered by human embrace. And so did I. As I held his upper body, it felt like I melted right into his heart. I thought about patients who had been hospitalized for long periods of time with no one to touch or hold them. The healing power of love; how their bodies must crave it, even if they aren't aware of it.

Needless to say, more loving medicine for Erik finally arrived; Jenny. She'd been gone since Day Five. It was almost two weeks since she'd seen him. And he didn't remember her being at the hospital at all. She peeked around the curtain into his room with that gorgeous smile. Sappy as it sounds, when their eyes met, it was all over, for all of us. Not a dry eye in the house or should I say the ICU.

Jenny has a huge soft spot tucked under her firecracker exterior. She took one look at him in all his ICU glory and said, "Aww...Baby," then stepped close to softly touch his face. Even the nurses peeked in, just to witness the tenderness and love that most of us take for granted on a daily basis. And of course, Erik's tear-filled eyes did the talking for him, just like Jenny said. She loved his eyes and how they spoke to her.

Date Night in ICU

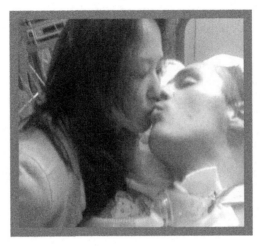

We all know that Jenny's presence would be the best thing for Erik. Everyone there held that presence with high regard and promptly gave them their privacy. The following day was a Saturday. A group of friends and family had congregated in the waiting room that evening when Jenny strutted in, dressed to the hilt. We were all taken by surprise, wondering why she was so dolled up. I asked if she was going out. She said, "Yes, I have a date!" My heart sank. I didn't have a clue what she really meant. "It's date night for Erik and me. We're going to watch movies!" The nurses in ICU had shanghaied a DVD player for Erik's room earlier that week because one of his friends brought him the movie, *Avatar*, one of Erik's favorites. So he and Jenny spent that evening together in ICU, watching movies. Most importantly, she held him. They didn't want her in his bed while he was in ICU, but she would sneak and snuggle up beside him whenever she could. Their relationship was so new, that none of us could imagine what the future would hold for them.

Some of Erik's friends were very protective of him. They didn't want to see him hurt if Jenny decided to end things. Erik was well aware of the harsh reality of his situation. He was also well aware that Jenny would need to make a choice about their relationship. But right at that moment, it was quite clear it didn't matter what was going to happen. They had *that moment*. It was a moment filled with love not words. And isn't that all any of us really have?

Erik's Facebook Wall Post to Jenny
(two months after the accident)

Erik Fugunt
The pain of standing beside me while I was struggling for life, knowing the odds were against me and that any moment could have been our last together were no doubt more difficult than anything I could ever imagine. To be completely honest it was the most devoted, kind, brave and selfless act I have ever had the honor to be a part of. Although I could only hear your voice, I want you to know that I fought for us and you are the reason I am here. I was, am, and forever will be yours. I love you and am in your debt for being so incredibly strong in my time of need. I pray every day that somehow someway I will get a chance to repay the courage, love and undying faith for our relationship that you have shown for it. I love you.
June 24, 2010 at 1:35pm

Legends of Wilmington

From the night Erik asked me to stay with him, I was with him nearly 24/7, only sneaking time during the day for a quick nap and shower. The nights were when he wanted me most, which became increasingly harder for me. Chairs and sleep don't cut it for me. I need to be horizontal. I was sleep deprived but I knew it would end. It was what Erik needed. And I know it was what I needed. Those weeks were grueling and filled with demanding negotiations between Erik and everyone; nurses, doctors, department heads and me. He went head to head with some people and I, of course, tried to be diplomatic.

He hated the feeding tube. He could feel that it was creating a groove in the skin around his nostril and was mad that it would likely be a permanent marking. It was shocking to me that he cared about a little thing like that when there were clearly more grave conditions to be concerned about. Maybe he figured that his handsome face was his best asset now. And he was still courting Jenny. So who knows? But hating that feeding tube may have driven his desire for solid food.

A few weeks after the accident, still in ICU, he insisted he could swallow around his tracheotomy. No one believed him but he created quite a ruckus. He got his way by convincing Doctor Mindy and Nurse Louise to let him eat solid foods, in spite of the tracheotomy and despite the staunch disapproval of the Respiratory Department.

He asserted himself, with or without the approval of authority. So the accident hadn't changed that. I recognized his fiery spirit and suddenly fostered a whole new appreciation of how he used it. Exhausting? Yes. Worth it? You bet, every precious challenging minute. It meant he was fighting; to live.

One afternoon I entered his room while he was asleep. His legs were uncovered and he was positioned in such a way that took my breath away. His eyes were closed. His lifeless legs were slightly bent and together at the feet. They looked just like Christ's legs when he was hung on the cross. I sat at the foot of his bed and wept, kissing Erik's feet. I prayed to Mary Mother of Christ, as I tasted a tiny grain of her torture and sorrow. How did she do it? How did she watch her son die? Could she help me now? Please Mary, find a way. Please help me.

Erik rarely slept at night. He wanted me nearby constantly. One night, he dozed off briefly. Thank God for a break. It was about 2 a.m. and I remember sneaking out of his freezing cold room and staggering to the Kona Café just down the hallway. I placed two bottles of cranberry juice at the cash register. I must have been a pitiful site; all bundled up in a jogging suit, a heavy brown sweater with a scarf wrapped around my head, tears of exhaustion dried on my face.

The cashier, a gentle young man, spoke kindly, "Don't worry ma'am. It's gonna get better." Then he paid for my juice and smiled. His kindness touched me so deeply. As I thanked him, my eyes filled up and I cried with humility as I stumbled down the hallway back to Erik's room, taking my familiar position at his feet. I held, massaged and kissed Erik's feet every chance I could get. I didn't realize he had used his cell phone to photograph me. I don't know how it made him feel, since he couldn't feel it physically. And I didn't ask. But he found it worthy of snapping a picture.

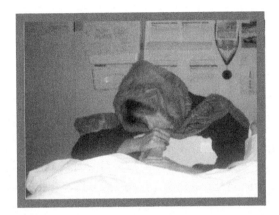

My faithful
ritual at
Erik's feet

It seemed like the male nurses always had the night shift. They were always very kind and comforting. There were three in particular, Brad, Aaron and Calvin that made a lasting impression. Those guys were incredible.

Aaron, the night nurse, would sit and chat with us. One night he told us about a guy he knew who had become a paraplegic after a motorcycle accident. This guy lived with his mother for a period of time after his accident. He became bitter and the demands he made on his mother became too much for her to take. One snowy night, this guy fell out of his wheelchair into the cold snow. He growled at his mother to get him up. She'd had enough of his terrible attitude. She walked to the house and told him to get himself up. He sat in the snow and stewed for a while, then began to laugh out loud. He picked himself up, brushed himself off and made it to the house by himself. From that moment he started to make a life for himself. He is now married and works as a mechanic on motorcycles. I'm sure he shared that story to help prepare us for the tough days ahead.

Nurse Calvin would talk about movies and bring his favorites for Erik to watch and Nurse Brad was just cool. Erik named him *The Master Stick,* because Brad could draw blood and insert IVs like no other. When someone would be struggling to stick Erik, he'd ask for *The Master*, Brad. Erik really liked those guys. I'm sure he could relate to them as peers and he held them in high regard.

When they would wash Erik and clean him after a bowel movement, they made light of it somehow to help ease Erik's humiliation and my helplessness. During those times, I wondered what was really ahead. How *were* we going to do this? I had to remind myself what I'd told Erik, "*with strength, determination and love*". That's how. That's the only game plan I had. So far, it was working and the nights spent with those amazing night nurses helped me believe in the game plan even more.

Ling was the friend that brought Erik the DVD of *Avatar*, a movie he loved. Since the nursing staff had worked their magic to surprise him with a DVD player in his room, that movie played 24/7. And I mean nonstop. Erik loved the movie prior to the accident, but now it held an even more succinct meaning for him. He could completely relate with the main character, who was a paraplegic. He could relate to the experience of walking again in a different dimension, of falling in love, of sacrifices and choices that would require him to maneuver through life in ways that he could have never imagined.

Watching the movie *Avatar* was an integral part of his healing process; the message, the music and the imagery, all powerful. His Facebook entry that follows will tell you how he felt about the movie when he saw it a few months before his accident.

Erik's Facebook

Erik Fugunt

AVATAR! Ok hmm.. trying to think of one word to describe this movie... LEGENDARY !!!!! The 3D was the most stunning visual experience you could ever imagine. Plot was epic and heart touching. Rate this movie? 10/10 no joke, it was that AMAZING!!! If you haven't seen it, take off work, skip school, miss church, whatever it takes to get there and see it in 3D. You will love it !!!

December 28, 2010 at 4:17am

Now Erik was beyond seeing the movie in 3D. As it played around the clock on a television screen in an ICU room, he was living it.

And since we're talking legendary, it's time you learn about Tom. One afternoon, about a week into ICU, two gentlemen dressed in suits and ties entered Erik's room. It took us by surprise, to say the least. "Suits and ties?" I'm thinking, "What the heck is this?"

Bill, the respiratory hero from the trauma team, had shared Erik's story with "*the suits*" so they wanted to meet him. Bill kept tabs on Erik. Everyone involved in that unbelievable trauma scene kept tabs on him. You might say he became the pet in the unit. So here were two white collar guys who wanted to know more about the Superman who survived against all odds. They greeted Erik and asked him what he would call all this; meaning what had happened to him and his progress. Erik didn't have an answer so after a few moments of silence, I spoke. "A miracle," I said and pointed to the symbol hanging on wall.

They both smiled and replied, "Amen to that."

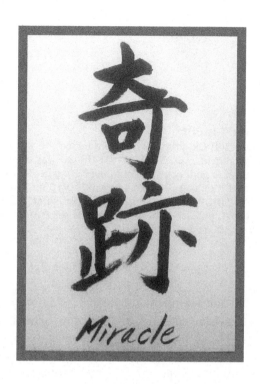

Miracle

"Miracle" - a symbol I hung
in Erik's ICU room

My curiosity was killing me so I was glad when Erik mouthed, "So, what do you guys do here?" Good question, since they weren't what he was used to seeing in the ICU. They introduced themselves as vice presidents of the hospital and wanted to know if there was anything they could do to make him more comfortable. Even though Erik still had the tracheotomy, he was getting quite adept at communicating past it and continued chatting with them for about ten minutes. Among other things, Erik communicated that the hospital had already done more for him than he could ever imagine. Before they left the room, they commented that perhaps his story could be shared with others as a source of hope, courage and strength. Erik graciously extended his services in whatever form they thought might be appropriate one day, then reached to shake their hands goodbye and thanked them for their concern and visit. That was our first encounter with the legendary VP Tom, our Superman of New Hanover Regional Medical Center – the man that would follow Erik closely and impact both of us profoundly as the weeks progressed. He was nicknamed Superman because he was...well...a super man. He always showed up at just the right time. He fixed any problem that we encountered. And he was just a great guy. The kind you want to have watching your back.

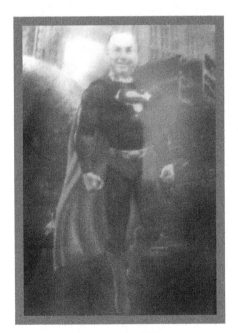

Superman aka VP Tom
framed as a parting gift for Erik

Photograph courtesy of New Hanover Regional Medical Center

I truly was amazed at the way Erik interacted with others. He was smooth. If he liked someone, he was delightful, charming and gracious, just as he had been with those two men in suits and many of the hospital staff. I knew his charming skills were in full bloom when he was able to convince Nurse Nikki that he could *bag* himself; manually pump the oxygen into his own lungs during a transport to an MRI.

When he didn't like someone, well, let's just say they knew it. And I was learning that I wanted to be more like that; more candid and bold, more genuine and care less about what others thought of me. I had a lot to learn from my son. And the lessons would continue with increasing intensity as the days rolled along.

The time had come for my friend, Lori, to return to Pittsburgh. Before she left we sat together in the car, in a parking lot outside the Verizon store where she'd driven me to pay Erik's cell phone bill. It's kind of crazy when you think about the mundane responsibilities that need tended to in the midst of the drama; bills to pay, college withdrawal, his banking, unemployment case file, tax returns and such.

Lori and I sat in the car, looked at each other in disbelief and then we cried, and cried, and cried. We'd been best friends for almost twenty years now, through thick and thin; not friends that talk or hang out together every day or even every week, just best friends with different lifestyles. Our common values and respect for each other seemed to be the glue that held us together so tightly for so many years. Our shared experiences of the past year had transformed that glue into cement.

So there we sat.

Her son was dead.

Mine was supposed to be dead, but was alive and paralyzed.

Good God, what was happening?

After we pulled ourselves together and reduced our crying to sighing sobs, we talked about the possibility that God had a plan for us. He damn well better have a plan because the burdens were getting to be too much. Our shoulders were tired and weary. We talked about the salon staff; how wonderful and supportive they were, but also how shaken up they must be. Their owner's son was killed 11 months ago and the former owner's son lay paralyzed in critical condition. They must have wondered how much more we could take and may have been nervous about the future of the salon and its leadership. Undoubtedly, I knew the salon would be a grounded healing place for both of us; an entity that epitomized our grit and commitment to each other. Yes, it was different now than when we started it; we were different too, inside and out.

But I took comfort in knowing that Lori would boldly keep forging ahead in spite of her grieving. I always believed in her, trusted her and counted on her. And although her grieving was taking its toll, I believed in her more than ever. I had to. I needed something strong to hold on to, my Rock. She headed for home, knowing that I'd be alright too; knowing we'd be there for each other like no one else could be.

Wounds — Past & Present

Erik's vice presidential visit was such a lift. It's exciting to be noticed, even if it is in a hospital bed, perhaps especially in a hospital bed. That visit seemed to hit Erik in a deep place; the place of recognition. You see, Erik had always been special, doing amazing things, but he always seemed to get into trouble with his talent, not use it for positive recognition.

I suppose when we, as parents would tell him how special he was, he figured we were biased; that all parents think that about their children. And I guess we do. Either way, recognition seems to have much more impact coming from a stranger; and a stranger wearing a suit and tie, well, need I say more? Erik's story may be able to inspire others, but the visit from Tom and his associate really bolstered my son's spirits as well, just what he needed to undergo the extensive spinal fusion that awaited him.

Erik was banking everything on that surgery, for a chance to walk again or at the very least, some improvement in function. We all were. Despite the neurosurgeon's certainty that he would never walk again, Erik instructed him to operate aggressively and give him the best chance he could. The T9 vertebra was shattered completely from the impact of Erik's back slamming into the tree, right about the place where the bottom of his book bag would have laid across his spine. A shard of that vertebra was wedged into the spinal column and Erik wanted it removed.

The neurosurgeon assured him that he would do the best he could, but never promised to remove the shard. I remember taking that man's hands and kissing them before he operated on my son.

From the stunned expression on his face, I'm guessing that no one had ever done that before. I'm sure that Erik's antics and my obscure behavior disrupted the normal hospital routine, hopefully for the better.

Obviously, in Erik's grave condition, attempts to repair his spinal injury at the onset were not a priority like we would have hoped. They never expected him to survive. And curtly stated, from the neurosurgeon's calculations, he was permanently and irreversible paralyzed. So there was no need to rush and fix his spine; not what we were thinking.

They used the term *severed* when they referred to his spinal cord. We thought of his cord as *pinched*; like a wedged rock that had pinched a rubber hose closed. We figured that if the rock (the shard of his T9) was removed, then the hose (his spinal column) would have a chance of allowing water (spinal fluid and nerve impulse) to flow again. We believed his body would find a way to heal itself if the passage was clear for it to do so. I'll never forget Erik telling me, "Mom, I know my body can regenerate. I know I can grow new nerve tissue. I know it. But not if there is a bone in the way."

He didn't need to convince me. I was on board completely. Our concept made perfect sense to us. And we figured the longer we waited to remove the shard, the more nerve endings would die. The neurosurgeon's goal was not the same as ours. His objective was to stabilize Erik's back with two titanium rods attached at his T6 and T12 vertebra, below and above the shattered vertebrae, without causing any more damage. But Erik held hope that he would also remove the cause of his paralysis. After fifteen days in Trauma ICU Room 8, Erik was wheeled to the PCU, Progressive Care Unit. His spinal fusion surgery was scheduled for the following day.

As a side note, I just have to say I had no idea what all the acronyms meant. ICU, PCU, LDI, ABC, XYZ. Those medical folks had an acronym for everything and they threw them around like baseballs at the park. Since it was their everyday language, I'm not sure if they forgot that not everyone knows what they are talking about or if they just like making you feel stupid. Either way, it was a struggle at times, just to follow the language.

While in ICU, Erik had undergone a procedure to place a filter in his inferior vena cava to help prevent blood clots from reaching his heart and lungs. Other than that procedure, MRIs, x-rays and CT scans, the spinal fusion was his first major surgery since the intensive lung surgery that had been performed almost two weeks ago. Now, the concern again, was for his lungs. Would they hold up for such a long surgery that required him to be in a prone position for six hours? If not, the doctors prepared us for a return trip to the ICU. If all went well, Erik would head back to his room in the Progressive Care Unit.

A few hours after Erik was transferred to PCU, my brother Terry, sister-in-law Luanne and niece Ashley arrived from Frogtown, Pennsylvania. Lucky for them, they missed the whole Trauma ICU scene. Even with all the personal touches I'd made to his ICU room, the gravity of that Trauma Unit felt like a doorstep to the cemetery. No wonder, ICU patients are like deer in hunting season, a lot of them don't make it *out of the woods* alive. The PCU had been recently renovated and felt more like a hotel than a hospital. There was a couch that converted to a bed so I was able to be horizontal instead of sitting in a chair when I tried to sleep. I say "tried" to sleep because it was literally impossible. Erik didn't sleep. At night, every fifteen minutes, I'd hear, "Mom?" And I'd be right there at his side, tending to whatever he needed.

Come to think of it, he didn't like to sleep when he was a little boy either. The feeling of exhaustion was hauntingly familiar. He always did keep me awake at night. Why should this be any different?

Needless to say, Erik was glad to see his family from Frogtown. He was almost weaned from his tracheotomy so voice communication was easier. He and his cousins, especially Ashley, who is three years his elder, played together often as children. During Erik's very early and formative years, we spent a lot of time at my family's farm in Frogtown. Erik's father, Ron, would arrive at the farm with some fun adventure in tow. Whether it was spelunking, motorbikes, boating, hang gliding or anything wild, there was never a dull moment when Uncle Ron and Cousin Erik were around. I guess things hadn't changed much.

Terry, Lu and Ash were glad to see him too, even though they had a rough time when it was time to suction Erik's tracheotomy and lungs. Terry would look down at the floor and Luanne would leave the room with a queasy stomach. But they hung in there like troopers and quickly adjusted. And thank God they did. I had no idea how much I would need their help with the hell that lie ahead.

Friday morning, April 30th, sixteen days after the crash, Erik was taken to surgery for placement of titanium rods in his spine. His father and I stayed in the preparation room with him as nurses, anesthesiologists and respiratory staff all prepared Erik for cuttin' time. I'll never forget how he interacted with a nurse who was rubbing Erik's hand, speaking to him with soothing words when tears started to well up in her eyes; she had a son of her own about that age and couldn't help but imagine him lying in that bed. That's when Erik gently took *her* hand. Holding it tightly, he said to her, "Don't worry, everything's gonna be okay. I'm gonna be alright."

Her eyes twinkled as a smile appeared on her face; a few of her tears spilled over. He'd done it again, pulled off one of those tender, charming moments with perfect timing. He was definitely Hollywood material. And I'm sure he'd even do his own stunts.

While waiting for the surgical knife that morning, Erik also spoke to his father about spending more time with his little brother, Nick, whose 14th birthday happened to be the exact same day as Erik's accident; poor kid. What a crappy birthday.

"Dad, you gotta do more with Nick," Erik advised. "Spend more time with him. It goes so fast and look what's happened to me." I was floored with the level of maturity Erik was demonstrating, even minutes before a critical surgery. I suppose the critical level of the situation was a catalyst that spawned his rapid maturation.

We were prepared for a minimum six hour surgery. I sat outside with my niece Ashley for most of that time. It was a beautiful sunny day. The feeling of sunshine on my body took me away for a while. The surgery, the accident; none of it seemed real. I loved having Ashley there. She could see Erik in a different way. "He'll be fine," she'd say convincingly. She sympathized and tended to him, but maintained remarkable composure. To watch her with him, you'd think that Erik was in the hospital to have his tonsils out. No big deal. She really rocked. And he was so glad to see her. He told her he'd make it to her wedding in four months. And she expected him to do just that.

The surgery required less time than expected, five hours, and according to the neurosurgeon, was successful. Ron and I spoke with him; he didn't remove the shard of bone that had severed the spinal column. He showed us pictures of the 12 inch long titanium rods he placed in Erik's back. Ron and I were both surprised at the length and curvature of the rods. It looked to us like the rods were curved forward at the top. The neurosurgeon explained that he bent the rods to accommodate the natural curvature of the spine.

Whatever? It looked odd to us but we didn't know a lot about human anatomy. We were just relieved that Erik made it through, that his lungs held up and he didn't need to go back to the ICU. We all waited for Erik in his room on the PCU floor. It was about 6:30 p.m. when we saw him coming around the corner on a transport table.

Ron went to his side immediately as they wheeled him into his room. "Just get away from me." Erik moaned in agony and shouted. "Just leave me alone." Oh my God, what had we done to him? I felt the blood in my face rush to my feet. The attendants told us that he was hard to keep sedated. They'd given him enough drugs to put down an elephant and he still wasn't out.

We all lingered in the hallway outside Erik's room for about half an hour, then one by one, we quietly entered his room. It was awful. Once he was able to tolerate our presence, he begged for help. That night was the hell I'd mentioned earlier.

Erik writhed in excruciating pain, his face horribly red and swollen from lying prone on his stomach for so many hours. Pain medication was being administered, but not fast enough or strong enough for him to feel relief. Oh my God, it was absolutely awful. There was nothing we could do. We'd brought the DVD and TV from ICU with us. So I played *Avatar*, hoping it would help distract him from his misery.

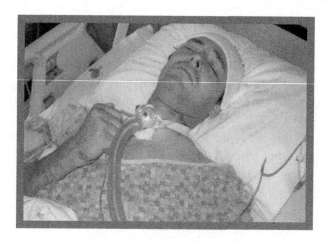

Erik, the day after his spinal fusion

His PCU nurse, Edwina was doing everything in her power to help. And I mean everything. "If we give him anymore drugs, we could overdose him. This kid has incredible tolerance; I can't believe it," she said under her breath. We'd just have to suck it up and tough it out.

"I can't stand it! Sit me up!" he'd command. We raised the back of his bed. "Higher." We raised it more. "Higher!" he shouted. We had him positioned straight up and down, as vertical as the bed would go. He looked like he was standing in bed and going to fall out. Oh man, what a sight. He was doped out of his mind, whooping and hollering along with the beautiful blue *Avatar* creatures as they chanted their war cry to defend their spectacular world. Erik lived in that world now; the land where the hero was a paraplegic who longed to walk again, the land where the paraplegic fell in love unexpectedly, the land where a battle must be fought and won to ensure survival, the land where life was part of a sacred connection, not part of an institution or government statistic. Sitting nearly upright in a hospital bed, whooping a war cry, his eyes wide and wild staring into mine, all I could do was join in. I put my hand to my mouth and pounded my lips to make my own sounds of battle cry. There we were, whooping it up together. Whatever it took, we had to get through the night.

Eventually, he shouted to be laid back down, crying and begging for help to relieve the pain. My heart was torn to shreds. Terry, Luanne, Ashley and Ron had to leave. I hadn't slept in over two days, but I knew I had to muster just one more night, for Erik's sake. I stayed awake all night to make sure he got his extra hit of Dilaudid – a derivative of Morphine – every six minutes, on top of the IV drip and oral medications that were being administered. It was absolutely numbing. I remember staring at the clock, counting off six minutes, religiously, from 11 o'clock that night to 7 o'clock the next morning.

About that time, Terry, Luanne and Ashley appeared, fresh and ready for duty. What a site for sore and tired eyes. I handed full duty to them so I could retreat to the Hospitality House for some sleep. I knew Erik was in good hands, in fact, the best of hands. Terry patiently repositioned Erik at least every five minutes and when Ashley got caught handling the Dilaudid drip, Erik defended her by telling the nurse he instructed her to hold it. Luanne tended to the many other demands of his barking. Seeing Erik in such pain and suffering was probably more taxing than the actual work of his caretaking. Both together were enough to drop me.

I slept about least four hours before I returned that afternoon to find them all working together like a finely tuned machine. Each one had their duty and they executed like soldiers. Erik of course, was the general, barking orders. It was quite enlightening. And the troops helped me convince Erik to drink prune juice since he hadn't moved his bowels in days.

General Erik would tell the troops to take a break and go see the sites in Wilmington. Luanne would emphatically tell him they didn't come to see Wilmington, they came to see him! They stayed by his side, faithfully, when he needed it most and when I needed it most. "That's what family is for," Luanne, my sister-in-law said over and over. For whatever reason, there were so many people in that hospital that didn't have the support or love of family with them. Living through this ordeal, I learned how wonderful my family really is and how lucky I am to have them.

The next day, my backup troops, Terry and Company had to return to their lives and Frogtown. Erik's pain was not in the screaming range anymore. Ashley told him to keep the pillow she'd brought for him and keep it he did. She'll never get it back. Erik insisted on getting a picture of them together. After he thanked them profusely for making the trip down to help out, he commended Uncle Terry on his patience and ability to reposition his body every five minutes to make him more comfortable.

I said a tearful goodbye at the elevator. It was hard; very hard. I knew my big brother wanted desperately to make it better for us, to keep helping us. I knew he was distraught.

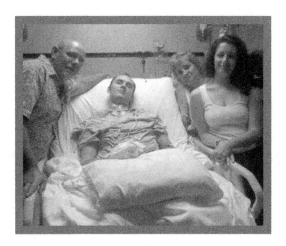

Terry, Luanne and Ashley with Erik
just before they went home

Both of my brothers must have imagined what they would do if it were their son that was in that situation, because their sons rode motorcycles too. I felt my big brothers' empathy. We had a hard time collecting ourselves, but we did. They stepped onto the elevator, the doors closed and that was that. I'd be okay. I knew that; deep in my gut. I work well independently; my grade school report cards said so.

If only I were that child again. Oh to go home and let Mom and Dad do all the work and let my body fall into bed with not a care in the world. How I wished to be small again and back in that safe place of my parent's care. Now it was my turn to provide that place for my adult child. I'd be flying solo again, as Erik's mom and advocate.

I was hoping to see Chuck again, soon. We spoke every day, but it's not the same as seeing his face. I was always preoccupied when we spoke on the phone, yet he continued to faithfully journal Erik's progress and patiently listened to me. No wonder I love him. And though Ron lived nearby and we had joined forces temporarily to get Erik through this, we were divorced for a reason; we were very different from one other.

For the first time since I'd been here, I felt very much alone, not lonely, just alone.

That evening, I went to tour the adjacent Rehab Hospital while Ron stayed with Erik. I have a hard time admitting this, but man, I was emotionally and physically cooked, burnt to a crisp. The visit to the Rehab left me with an even deeper pit in my stomach. Before I returned to Erik's room, I stopped by the Hospital Chapel with the woman that took me on the tour. It was a much needed visit to the quietness of reverence.

I collapsed in the presence of God and crumbled in front of the woman that took me on the tour. I was embarrassed that she saw me on my knees, sobbing and whimpering like a little puppy lost in the wilderness. It was okay for God to see me in my weakness; but it was not okay for her to see me that way. I realized that I wanted to be alone – with God. Reality was setting in. Our lives had been shattered. There was no way to escape it. No way to spin it. My inner cheerleader was saying, "Keep fighting, Erik! You can win! You can triumph over this situation!"

In my heart, I believe in the healing gifts of massage, energy, prayer and love. I believe in miracles. I believe in biomechanics and modern medicine. I believe Erik will walk again one day. But my inner child was saying, "I'm so frightened. I'm so tired. I don't know what to do. I can't fix it."

Within the safety of that tiny hospital chapel I was able to admit my helplessness, to God and to myself. Who am I to expect, even demand that Erik be healed? Why believe in any of that stuff? No answer came, only silence. And isn't that faith, believing in what you can't explain?

> *"Now faith is the assurance of things hoped for,*
> *the conviction of things not seen."*
> Hebrews 11:1

I did my best to put on the face, wipe my tears, suck it up and get back to Erik's room. By the time I returned, Ron had gone and I was greeted by Erik in the most angry, hostile manner. "I wanna know, Mom. I wanna know," he verbally attacked me. "Did you know Frank before you left my dad? Just tell me the truth. I wanna know. Did you leave my dad for Frank?"

Where the heck did that come from? I almost fell over! Already on the verge of collapse from complete exhaustion, with only a few hours of sleep over the past four days, I was totally blindsided. Here was my son, lying in a hospital bed, paralyzed, injured beyond the boundaries of imagination and he furiously jumps me about Frank. I'd had a serious relationship with Frank, a pseudo twelve year marriage actually, after I left Erik's father seventeen years ago.

When Frank and I parted ways, our communication waned but I did receive a text from him when he learned of Erik's accident, saying he was keeping us in his prayers and that Erik was a tough kid and would make it through this. Erik and Frank always butted heads. I knew there was resentment on Erik's behalf, I just didn't know how deeply seeded it was. I was already at the end of my rope. I felt myself letting go and I fell to a place of anger. My face felt red hot. I was red hot. I didn't think. I just let go. I'd have to sink or swim in my anger.

I got mad, really mad and explained that I did not leave his father for Frank; I left for me. He insisted that I must be lying because I was so mad and defensive. "Damn right I'm mad!" I went on. "This isn't important! My son is lying in a hospital bed in critical condition and I'm defending myself *again* over something that didn't even happen!"

"Well, everyone said it happened that way," Erik ensued. He mentioned certain people that reinforced this theory of the divorce.

Needless to say, I was pissed and on top of that I was feeling horribly guilty about being pissed, a double whammy from my inner critic who was gaining power due to my weakened state of exhaustion. "Not that it's any of your business, Erik! What happened with your father and me is between your father and me. But to clear the air once and for all, I did not leave your father for Frank! You and anyone else can believe whatever you like. Sometimes people have to believe things that aren't true because they can't make sense of anything else."

I told him how I'd met Frank; he was one of the guys that my friend rounded up to help me move out of the home that Ron and I had built together. I had expected to date a certain guy, very much unlike Frank, after I left his father. But that never happened. My voice boomed like that of a famous movie line. "You wanna know the truth? That's the truth. At this point, I have nothing left to lose and neither do you."

Erik retorted, "Well maybe you'd have been better off with that certain guy who wasn't like Frank." Regardless of how Erik felt about my choices, I left his dad carrying my own guilt ridden baggage. When I divorced Ron, I promised myself *and* God that as my punishment, I would never ever marry again. It took me seventeen years and a recent conversation with my Pastor Sam to finally accept forgiveness and consider a marriage with Chuck. Chuck had even asked for Erik's approval to marry me and it was graciously given. Erik liked Chuck. Chuck wasn't like Frank and he wasn't like Ron. He was a softie and Erik called him the voice of reason. But Chuck's name was never mentioned during this heated confrontation. He wasn't part of this wound.

We chewed around a bit longer, tit for tat, this for that. Erik's wheels were turning. Even though he was heavily medicated, I could tell that he was thinking about his future and the tough choices that were ahead. "That's what women do. They leave you for another man. And then they lie about it. That's just what happens. How do I know that won't happen again?" Erik stated.

Obviously the break up with his former girlfriend was part of this rage as was his concern for the future of his relationship with Jenny. I didn't have any good answers. There were no good answers or guarantees. I only tried to assure him that's not always how it works.

Then it was oddly quiet for a while. Clearly we had ventured into some deep tender territory. Not only were we battling present wounds, the horrific wounds of the past had surfaced as well. As the minutes ticked by, I realized all I could do was be present in the horrible, awkward, ugliness. If any healing were to come of it, it would come from grace, on its own accord and not from any words I spoke.

As I sat there beside him, I began to sob. I was so sad. I was so humbled. I felt like the one who had really screwed things up. I cried and cried. I told him how sorry I was that I wasn't there to keep him safe. I kept sobbing, "I'm so sorry, Erik. I'm so sorry." Erik wasn't crying. He told me that he and his dad were all cried out. The PCU nurse was astutely aware of the heavy but delicate situation. While tactfully respecting our privacy, she offered to get us both some hot tea and delivered it with a kind smile. I was impressed with the graciousness demonstrated so many times by the hospital staff. They recognized and respected the full scope of healing. The precious process of healing wounds, past and present, the natural process of healing the body and the soul, was in full swing, for both of us.

As we sat together quietly in the serene aftermath of the cleansing storm, Erik said, "Mom, I felt my right leg move. I moved it." I lifted the blanket and watched as I asked him to do it again. He couldn't. But I believed him. I believed his nerve endings were fighting, struggling to survive, just like he was.

A few weeks later, Erik made this comment out of the blue. "Mom, you wouldn't be able to tolerate Dad." I knew what he meant. He was able to see our differences from an adult viewpoint now, instead of the little boy who was wounded. It was his way of conveying that even though he wished we could have stayed together as a family unit, he was accepting the fact that we weren't.

I responded, with no malice whatsoever for his father, "No I wouldn't and your dad wouldn't be able to tolerate me either honey." There was a nod of understanding, from his head and his heart.

I found out later that Erik made an impromptu visit to see Frank about four months after his accident. I don't know the details of the visit, just that it was good. I don't really need to know the details. It's none of my business at this point. It's theirs. I'm just glad that Erik made the visit and that he has found peace with that situation.

Now I could see that we were coming full circle. This whole scenario was like a do-over of our entire life together. Erik's accident had taken us through all the stages of his life from birth to early adulthood. When he was in ICU, it was like he was born all over again. He required the same care as an infant; from feeding to bowel movements to being held. Then as he progressed, he became more demanding, just like his preschool years, keeping me up 24/7. Now we'd arrived at the age when his father and I divorced. All those wounds were surfacing. Each stage of his recovery correlated closely with each stage of his childhood. And we weren't done yet.

Code Blue

"What woman in
her right mind
would want to
be with a man
who lies in his
own shit?"

Honest words
spoken by a broken
young man.

Apparently the prune juice that I insisted he drink for the last two days finally kicked in. I was reminded of a time when he was three years old. He would not go to the toilet to have a bowel movement. He would soil his pants and then giggle when I would change him. During one of those unnecessary episodes of changing him, when he began to giggle, I got the mess on my hands. I remember being so frustrated with him that I dabbed his mess on his own nose and said, "There! If I have to get messy from your dirty pants, so do you! How do you like it?" Well, his shitty grin quickly turned into a shitty wailing. He cried for a few moments until I cleaned his nose as well. After that, he didn't soil his pants again. Until now.

What woman would want to be with a man who lies in his own shit? I didn't know how to answer. Erik was faced with the humiliation of the loss of bowel control along with everything below his belly button. I was glad to see that it still mattered to him. It was a good sign that his integrity was intact and I hoped that pride would motivate him to work to manage his bowel function. But it was so scary. The nurses insisted that he would learn how to manage things; that Rehab would teach him a bowel program that would allow him to lead a normal daily life. That just sounded ridiculous and crazy to me, but I went along with it and encouraged Erik in concert with the nurse's voices. "We'll get it figured out, Erik."

Some of the people that had worked on Erik in the Emergency Room, but hadn't seen him since, visited him in his PCU room with disbelief. They were amazed at what they saw. They told Erik about the ER situation and what he looked like then. They also said that the week of Erik's accident they had three traumas involving young men and motorcycles and that Erik was the only one to survive.

When we were alone, later that morning, Erik said, "Mom, look at my left foot. I think it's moving. I think I can move it." Since I was constantly rubbing his feet anyway, I was right on it. I watched closely. Nothing. I continued to watch. Then I saw it. I saw his left foot move outward about one inch. I swear to it. I never saw it again after that.

I don't know what enabled it to happen; Erik's will power combined with some random nerve endings in his spinal column that were struggling to survive, or what. But I know what I saw. Erik felt and saw it too. He said it took every ounce of everything he had to do it. You could see his body collapse in exhaustion afterward.

After the momentous occasion of his tracheotomy removal, the Rehab evaluation team arrived in Erik's PCU room on a Monday morning, three days after his spinal fusion and nineteen days since the accident. They held him up in a sitting position and he made a lame attempt to brush his teeth. Look closely, you'll see a toothbrush sticking out of his mouth. He looked like hell.

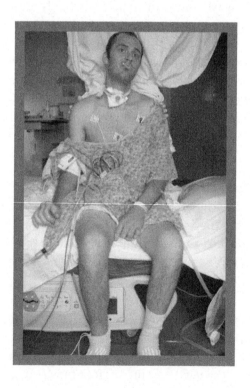

Erik sits up
held from behind
by a therapist

three days after the
spinal fusion

In retrospect, no wonder he looked like hell. He'd been through it.
I think of those who whine about a common cold for nineteen days. At
that time, every day felt like a life time, so I didn't have any concept of
his rapid progress. Nineteen days then was like nineteen lifetimes. Even
though this place in his recovery was scary, it was beginning to feel like
we were almost *out of the woods*.

He kept begging for a shower, bartering up a storm with the nurses, but
a shower was still not in the scope of his abilities. His balance was
nonexistent. Shower time would come soon though, because they said
he was ready for Rehab.

The next day, a young male therapist basically manhandled Erik into a
standard wheelchair. The head therapist that was spotting Erik was a
staunch, tough young woman. I'm glad she was there to spot him
because with Erik's poor balance, he flopped forward, only to land face
first into her bosom! Her face turned ten shades of red and her rigid
Stalin-like style was shattered. She gasped, "In all the years I've been
doing therapy, that's never happened."

"I'm so sorry!" Erik's charm and quick wit were ready and waiting.
"Well, at least I had airbags." A master of dry humor, he delivered
perfectly and we were all laughing hysterically.

All hopped up on Dilaudid, Erik wheeled himself from the 7th floor PCU
to the 1st floor Trauma ICU. He wanted to visit his intensive caretakers
to thank them and see the unit from a view other than laying on his
back. He was ornery and stubborn, insisting that he wheel the chair by
himself. And honestly, he looked like a super hero the way he navigated
and used his own strength to get around.

While all this is happening, I'm thinking to myself. "He just had his spine
fused a few days ago and he's doing this? I'm not so sure this is a good
idea."

Obviously, the illusionary power of Dilaudid was at work. On the way back to the 7th floor PCU, he began to fade and finally accepted some assistance from me. Upon his return, he was transferred to a regular room on the 5th floor of the hospital. Off we went, using the TV cart from the ICU as our moving van. It was loaded with all his stuff. And believe me; he was acquiring a lot of stuff. It looked like he had moved in. Well, I guess he had.

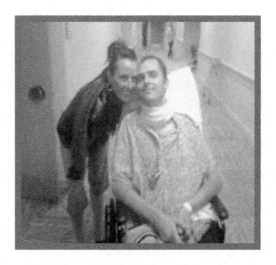

Erik's first wheelchair excursion, three days after the spinal fusion

I didn't bother settling in to this new regular hospital room. Erik would only be there for one day and night. And soon after getting there, the aftermath of pain from his wheelchair escapade to the ICU began to set in. As the night went on, it got worse. Everything got worse. I'd bounced back somewhat from hitting rock bottom a few days before, but I was in no way prepared for yet another night from hell. And I thought the worst was over. Nope, not yet.

It was late, almost midnight. I was bundled up in my blankets and nestled in the guest chair for the evening. *Avatar* played on the DVD player. Moans began to drone from the hospital bed that held my son. As minutes passed, Erik's moaning got louder and more persistent. I started getting seriously concerned. He began crying, from pain, both physical and emotional.

"I want my legs back, Mama. I want my legs back. I want a do-over. Please, please just give me that one day back. Just that one day, please. I want my legs back, Mama." Rivers of tears rolled down the sides of my son's face.

It was the one request that I couldn't bequeath. I prided myself on getting things done. I could orchestrate logistical tasks and have them done before anyone even thought of a deadline. You can't imagine how crushing and humbling it was for me to say through my stream of tears, "Me too. Me too, honey. I wish I could do that. I wish I could get that day back for you, Erik. I wish I could." There was nothing I could do; nothing anyone could do.

The pain and sorrow of real life, defining moments; we were being riddled with them like a steady flow of ammunition from enemy camp machine guns. When would it stop? Erik had held his ground. We needed a break. But war doesn't schedule breaks.

About midnight, Erik began to moan and writhe so badly with physical pain that I was literally standing with my face just inches from his. I made steady direct eye contact with his distant stare and commanded him, "Erik, hold on. You can do it. Hold on. I'm getting you some help."

"I can't do it, Mom." his voice faded along with his eyes as they began to roll back into his head. It scared the crap out of me. Suddenly, it felt like we'd stepped back *into the woods*.

"Erik!" I shouted as I held his eyes open with my fingers, "Erik, stay with me. Hold on." I thought we were losing him. I'd called for assistance a few minutes ago and no one had appeared yet.

So I looked at the wall above his head and hit the most logical button - a red button labeled **Assist**. Well Hi Dee Ho! The troops came a' running! Within seconds, eight nurses were in the room. "We need help," I pleaded with desperation. I didn't realize they all arrived so quickly because a Code Blue registered when I hit the red **Assist** button. When I saw them all take a huge sigh of relief, I realized they had rushed to service a Code Blue. "Sorry, but it said '**Assist**' and we need assistance – now! I think we're losing him." Erik found the little incident a bit humorous as a quick smirk snuck out between agonizing moans. One nurse asked the old familiar question. "What's your pain level on a scale from 1 to 10?"

"TWENTY!" yelled Erik. He got another straight IV drip of Dilaudid. I stayed awake all night watching him, in and out of lucidness. Once, during that long dreadful night he looked over at me and tearfully murmured, "Mom, I was walking. I dreamed I was walking. It was so real. I didn't want to wake up."

"It was real Erik. You are walking. In some dimension, like the dimension of *Avatar*, I assure you, you are walking. Never forget that." And I meant every word, with all my heart. As I watched him throughout the night, I wondered how he would ever function without the IV drip of pain killers. Was he already addicted? It had been almost three weeks of it. Or were his injuries so bad that his pain should be unbearable?

"Dah," I answered myself silently. His unbelievable tolerance shadowed the obvious. This guy was totally and literally smashed up. By now we had the full laundry list; shredded left lung, respiratory failure, cardiac arrest, pneumonia, multiple surgeries, broken left scapula, severely bruised left shoulder, eight completely shattered ribs, bruised heart, broken left hand, smashed vertebrae, severed spinal cord, fractured pelvis, sprained ankle; you know, just what you can expect when slammed against an oak tree at high speed – bodily destruction. When the sun rose the following morning, I whispered a prayer of thanks. Erik made it through the night, and so did I.

Until this time, the catheter for urination had been left in for the most part and attended to by nurses. Not anymore. That morning, my son had his first lesson in self-catheterization, the equivalent to adult potty training. He had no trouble with the logistics of the process, but he had lots of trouble accepting the fact that he had to do it. The former luxury of just whipping it out and pissing on a tree now seemed ever so sweet.

That afternoon, Erik made a heartfelt phone call to the man and wife, Don and Kay who lived at the scene of the accident, to thank them for staying with him until he was taken away by ambulance. They would later visit with Erik in Rehab and share encouraging words of wisdom. So many amazing people had been mysteriously and strategically placed in the wake of this tragedy; it was our responsibility to recognize them.

Then Nikki, a favorite nurse of Erik's from ICU, quietly entered his room. Even though she was a woman of few words, her mannerisms revealed her inner strength. She was the kind of person that got the job done with no nonsense. But Erik had managed to reach her heart too. Of Asian descent, she said to him in broken English, "I just want to tell you, after I see all you go through, it make me want to keep trying too." She'd been having some personal struggles of her own. I guess she and Erik had talked about them during his stay in ICU. He reached out to hug her and said, "Tell you what. You keep trying and I'll keep trying." They sealed the deal with tears. It all seemed surreal. The past three weeks brought one unbelievably touching moment after another, like rapid fire.

By late afternoon, orders came through to take Erik to the adjacent Rehabilitation Hospital. He didn't want to go. "I'm not ready," he pleaded. "I can't move. I can't do it. I'm not healed yet." The jaunt in the wheelchair yesterday had left him shell shocked with pain all night long. He didn't want to repeat another night like that, nor did I. "I can't do it. I'm not ready," He pleaded again.

I agreed with him at some level. He was one cracked up kid and because of his amazing recovery thus far, I was concerned that they were pushing it. But I sided with the doctors and told him we'd deal with it in Rehab. I promised him he wouldn't have to do anything he didn't want to. One bargaining chip we used was that the physiatrist in charge of Rehab was a pain management specialist. He'd be able to get Erik's pain under control. And he did. He ordered a pain patch that's used for terminal cancer patients. I think it was called Torodol. A 75 mg patch of that and oral medication of three to four Oxycodone every four hours helped Erik press on. It took about five days more before Erik actually made it out of his rehab room to begin slight, but measurable, rehabilitation.

The transport from the regular room to the Rehab was directed by a man named Manley. He took a shine to Erik immediately. A fellow motorcycle rider, they shared stories and made small talk. Erik instructed Manley to move ever so gently while he pushed the transport bed through the hospital corridors to the adjacent Rehab Hospital. Manley complied with compassion and moved ever so gently. He knew Erik was in horrible pain. I was moved by Manley's personal touch and commitment. He was the head of transport and came to move Erik because everyone else was busy, another drop of God's goodness. Manley faithfully visited Erik in Rehab, almost daily for the next five weeks.

The legendary VP of Operations, Tom aka Superman, the suited man that Erik met in ICU, also visited almost daily. I'm not sure the staff liked the VP visitation all that much. Erik would get chided about being a pet and receiving special attention. I felt like I was connected to the main pipeline of accountability and tried not to abuse the privilege. But there were a few times when I took Tom up on his continuing offer to, "Just call me if you need *anything*. I mean it." So when failed requests to fix Erik's shower through the regular chain of command failed, I called Tom. It was fixed immediately. If he wasn't able to handle a request, he directed me to the person that could. Tom became family to me during that time.

A few days after Erik entered rehab, I used the gift of two-hundred dollars that my Frogtown church collected for us and went shopping to get him sweatpants and t-shirts to wear for his therapy sessions. It's not like he worked up a sweat during therapy. But he did perspire profusely while lying in bed. And he went through a lot of sweat pants due to his inconsistent self-catheterization habits. I returned from Target, excited to find him in the bathroom with his dad. They used what I called the *hydraulic horse harness*, the lift, to hoist Erik out of bed and into a waterproof wheelchair that was also a toilet chair. Maybe those nurses were right after all. Maybe he could train his bowels. Halleluiah, after three weeks; he had a bowel movement on the toilet; even if it did require suppositories, patience and manual finger extraction. And best of all, he was finally getting that shower he'd been begging for. Woo Hoo! He was in there for an hour. He was starting to resemble a real person again. And that night, he slept a little bit, for real.

During the five weeks in Rehab, he was obsessed with the tweezers, picking at his own zits, body hair and scabs constantly. Having a few of my own chin hairs, I joined him in his activity. I'd say, "Hey, can you get this for me? I have trouble seeing up close." He'd zero in on my chin with precision. He even convinced me to let him tweeze a rogue eyelash from the inside corner of my eye. I don't think that hospital will ever have another patient quite like Erik. He was even trying to convince a nurse to let him pick at her face. What a riot; never a dull moment.

He was also a good sport about people practicing their blood drawing skills. He let one young fellow try sticking him about six times until he said, "Okay, you're done. Go get someone good, like *The Master*, Brad." It was amazing. Erik could actually *feel* the needle penetrate his vein. When he told a nurse just that, she said, "That's impossible. No way. You can't feel something like that." So Erik tested her. She stuck him once and he said she missed. He was right. She stuck him again and he said she missed. He was right again. She stuck him a third time. He said, "You got it." She disagreed. "No I missed again," she said. He insisted further, "I'm tellin' ya. You got it. Just try to draw some blood back."

Sure enough, blood filled her syringe. He stared at her with a smug look; one eyebrow raised and said matter-of-factly, "Told ya. I can feel it."

On Rehab weekends, Jenny came and stayed with Erik. I would normally sleep in the extra bed in Erik's room but on weekends, I received respite. Bless that little heart of Jenny's. She would curl up beside him in that hospital bed. At that point, no one ever stopped her. Erik even insisted that the extra bed be parked right next to his when she was there, making it feel like a double bed.

Again, Jenny's presence was the most instrumental factor in Erik's progress. During the week, when she was home in Mebane working, he would have a pining look in his eyes. On weekends, he couldn't get enough of her. I came into the room late one Saturday evening to find them curled up together in a tender quiet moment. I walked close to them to see if they were sleeping. She looked up at me and said, "Oh Mom, I'm so glad you're here." They had just watched a sentimental movie, *Family Man.* I sensed they were lingering in the emotional aftermath. I leaned over them and held them both for what seemed like a long time. As I held them, an image of Mary, Mary Magdalene and Jesus came to me. When Erik was still in ICU, I took him and Jenny on a guided mediation together to a special place of Light. This time, in an instant, they took me to a special place. I knew in my gut that this moment of love and tenderness resembled the relationship of that Holy Trio. I saw it. I felt it. I breathed deeply to store that precious fleeting moment of heaven into my cellular being.

But not all the moments were that precious. Erik navigated Rehab the same way he navigated ICU, with a combination of charm, defiance and feistiness that either infuriated or endeared whomever he was working with. He appeased me most of the time and agreed to take the barrage of supplements I gave him, but refused the doctor recommended protocol of Lovenox shots to prevent blood clots and other medications. When he asked me what my opinion was on the matter of refusing the Lovenox, all I could tell him was to listen to his body.

He insisted that particular medication made him feel light headed. He figured since he'd made it through the accident, if a blood clot was going to take him out, then so be it. And since I was constantly massaging his legs, he figured his blood was flowing more than the average sedentary patient. At any rate, he ticked off doctors and nurses. Of course, he had his favorites too, in photos that follow.

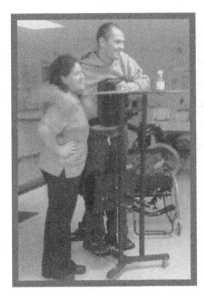

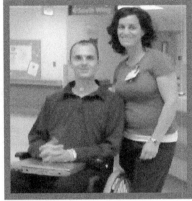

Left: Physical Therapist, Amber whom he playfully nicknamed Little Hitler

Right: Occupational Therapist, Noa

We didn't get pictures of all his favorites, like Tommy, his movie hookup; Joe, his nurse assistant and right-hand man; Marilyn, his wonderful massage therapist; Manley, his transporter; and of course VP Tom, his Superman; and let's not forget Chef Pete who made sure that Erik got the food he requested. There were so many people who did so much for both of us, more than I can mention.

The gentleman, Rick, that first held Erik's head still at the scene of the accident, made an unexpected visit to Erik at the Rehab Hospital. He'd heard through the grapevine that Erik had survived and wanted to see for himself. I met Rick for the first time in the hallway just outside Erik's room. "I could tell that you're his mother," he said. "He looks just like you."

"Not really," I said quizzically. "He must have had his helmet on when you were with him and all you could see were his eyes. His girlfriend says he has my talking eyes."

"Yes, that's right. His helmet was on," he said. "Well, he certainly does have your eyes." Rick shared how he stayed with Erik that morning, under the tree of impact. He talked about an unexplainable sense of peace that fell upon the accident scene during those first moments of the crash. He almost seemed unnerved as he spoke. It was obvious how profoundly affected he was when he described how peaceful it felt, especially in light of the violent crash that had just occurred.

I asked if he thought it was heavenly. He couldn't say. He couldn't describe the peacefulness, other than unbelievable and something he has never experienced before. That's what I call heaven on earth. He visited with Erik for a while, like everyone else, offering kind words of encouragement. Erik thanked him, for being there, now and then.

A few weeks after Erik entered the Rehab Hospital, the neurosurgeon who placed the rods in Erik's spine visited to check on Erik's progress. That discussion didn't go so well. Erik was downright pissed that the shard of bone wasn't removed from his spinal column.

I was disappointed as well. We grilled the neurosurgeon, not understanding why he didn't even try. He was becoming frustrated with us as well. I asked him to pretend that we were in kindergarten and to use language that we could understand.

Basically, he felt the attempt at removing the shard posed more risk of harm than potential good. I could see the anger burning inside of Erik. He was thankful that the neurosurgeon did the best he could. It just wasn't good enough.

One afternoon, I took a walk to the ER, to try and envision what had taken place there when my son was brought in. There was an empty emergency response vehicle at the door. I approached the EMS attendant with polite inquiries. She showed me the inside of the truck, where Erik would have ridden and how the workers would have hovered over him.

This person had heard about Erik's accident from the actual paramedics that worked on him and was shocked that he was still alive, let alone in Rehab. It was extremely sobering and emotional at the same time. Because of HIPAA laws, I wasn't able to procure the names of those who actually worked on Erik in the ambulance from her, but I knew someone who could; Superman!

Sure enough, Tom arranged for us to meet with the firemen and the EMS team, Linsay and Ben, who responded to the scene of the accident that day. My parents from Frogtown were fortunate enough to be present when we met the EMS team.

What an unbelievable experience it was, for all of us. The emergency responders thanked us for asking to meet with them. I guess they don't get that kind of request too often, maybe ever. They all said that they were just doing their job.

Truthfully, I think for them, meeting people like Erik was a part of their job they had been robbed of. I wanted them to know what a difference they make in the lives of others, just by doing their jobs and how it had impacted our lives in the most profound way possible. They were the first soldiers that responded to the 911 call, to save Erik's life. Their call of duty was one that I'll never be able to properly thank them for, ever.

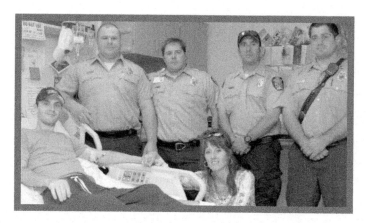

Erik, me, and the responding fireman

Photographs courtesy of New Hanover Regional Medical Center

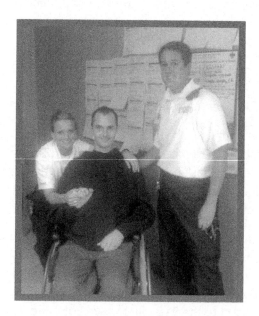

Erik with the responding paramedics, Linsay and Ben

Now we'd met all the folks that we could, who were involved along the way. The picture was complete. Each person of the story gave a special part of themselves to create a beautiful mosaic of life-saving proportion; a mosaic that I will hold dear and revere for the rest of my life. It's the reason I'm writing this book because the mind fails us over time and needs reminded of what the heart has stored so deeply.

After meeting with the emergency responders, I was numb from emotional overload. My parents and I returned to the Hospitality House for some quiet time. My mother and father, aka Poonie and Papa Hook, had driven all the way from the farm in Frogtown, Pennsylvania to spend a few days with their hospitalized grandson, and also to take care of me. So, of course, my mother insisted on cooking something. She looked through the kitchen cupboards of the Hospitality House and conjured up the perfect meal – tomato soup and buttered crackers. The three of us sat down together at the table, held hands and gave thanks. That meal was sacred because it was made by my mama; and I was a broken little girl that needed the comfort of her mama's love, just as I needed the stable reassurance of my father's hand.

It took some time for my father to gain his composure when he first saw Erik lying in the hospital bed, paralyzed. But after observing Erik's familiar spunk for a few days, he said, "I think just stay out of his way and he'll be fine." To this day, my father gets sick to his stomach when he hears the sound of a motorcycle. But in that hospital, he reassured me that everything would work out, even as he was suffering from his own undiagnosed neurological problem. Ten months later, my father was diagnosed with Non-Hodgkin's B Cell Lymphoma and Chronic Inflammatory Demyelinating Neuropathy causing paralysis in his legs. Since then, he has recovered but still undergoes monthly treatments. But when he visited Erik in the hospital, he was experiencing the onset of paralysis in his own legs – an interesting coincidence, to say the least. So he and Erik helped each other. Papa used the wheelchair as support when he took Erik to the hospital coffee shop. And Erik insisted that Papa use his leg compression devices to help with blood circulation.

Poonie brought homemade heating pads filled with corn and rice to place over Erik's broken shoulder and ribs. She brought him homemade cookies and candy too. I laughed out loud when Erik said, "Boy, that Poonie sure does know how to make a man happy." Apparently I wasn't the only one that felt the love in my mother's domestic gestures. And since I'd been monitoring Erik's meals to exclude any sugar, he'd hit the jackpot of sweets when she arrived. Papa Hook told Erik that Poonie had saved his life, once upon a time, way back when. And when he met Jenny, he told Erik that it looked like he had a good woman, one that saved his life too.

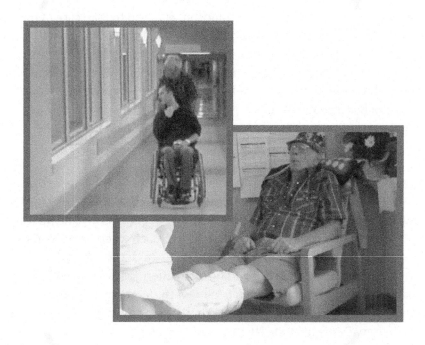

Top: My father, my son, each giving and receiving
Bottom: Papa naps with Erik's leg compressors

As the days turned into weeks, Erik would wistfully say, "I miss my legs. I just want them back," or "I just want to pee on a tree again, like I did before." He dogmatically resisted the catheter. When I'd place the heated rice bag on his abdomen to relieve the pain from his broken ribs, he'd urinate. So we thought maybe we could train his bladder to work with heat stimulation. It didn't work consistently. And he hated waking up in a wet bed, so eventually he gave in and began self-catheterization every four to six hours, just like the nurses instructed him to do.

A stranger walked into Erik's room one day. He quietly introduced himself as Reggie. It turned out that Reggie had been a former patient at this very Rehab Hospital. He too, had survived a devastating and tragic accident; one that left him paralyzed; one in which his beloved wife did not survive. His losses were beyond horrendous. But bottom line, Reggie had taught himself to walk again. He was a walking paraplegic – a contradiction of terms, indeed, but true. He could not feel his legs but he could walk. It was hard to believe. Doctor Liguori was Erik's physiatrist at the Rehab Hospital. He was also the physiatrist at the Rehab a few years back when Reggie miraculously "walked" out of there. Doctor Liguori had asked Reggie to stop and visit with Erik and another young man, Patrick, who was a patient that we'd met during our stay. Patrick's injury had come from helping move a deck into a pickup truck. It fell on his neck and he was an instant quadriplegic. He and Erik seemed to balance each other out. Erik shared his feistiness and Patrick shared his gentleness. And Reggie shared as much of his own life experience as he could, with both of them. He gave them the "inside scoop" of the rehab game. He shared messages to heal the soul, because according to Reggie, that's where healing begins. The mind and body follow. I couldn't agree more.

Reggie could "see" red in Erik's energy field; the anger. Not only could he see it, he knew firsthand what that anger was all about. And he knew it would be the first obstacle to Erik's recovery. He could also "see" how good Jenny's presence was for Erik and encouraged that relationship by having very candid conversations with her regarding life with a paraplegic.

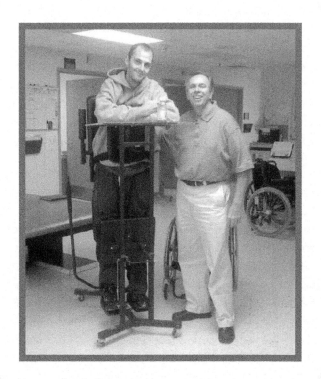

Reggie with Erik using the
standing frame for the first time

I didn't want to acknowledge Erik's intense anger, but I knew it was there. He'd say, "I hate my legs. They won't listen to me."

I'd respond, "That's okay. I'll love them for you," and continued to massage them nightly. I'd make him use whatever he could muster from his stomach muscles to move his legs in and out from a flexed position. He was getting thoroughly sick of me so I tried to wean myself away from him, taking walks at the park or on the beach.

On one such day, I drove to Wrightsville Beach, just minutes from the hospital, for a meditative walk. I parked and went into the market a few feet away for some change for the parking meter. When I returned to put money in the meter, I'd already been issued a $50 parking ticket.

I spotted the meter lady and ran to catch her, explaining how I was just there on break from the hospital to take a walk. I told her I was from out-of-town and of Erik's accident and that I didn't have change for the meter so I went into the market to get some. She had just left a few young surfers go, as they were making their way back to their expired meter, so I figured she would be cool about it. Wrong. She told me I'd have to go to the office and plead my case there. I literally dropped to my knees right there in the middle of the quiet street. "The office? Where is this office? You're kidding me right?" I was shocked at her cold shoulder and could feel myself starting to cry.

"No," she said. "There's nothing I can do." I picked my sorry-self up off that street and shook my head in disgust. Tears started to escape my infuriated eyes. As I walked away, with a defiant attitude, I turned back to her, "Really?" My sassiness stepped up to bat to keep my tears at bay. "Ma'am, do you have children?"

"Yes, two daughters," she answered.

I didn't miss a pounding step as I continued to march back to my car, exuding a wave of fierce disgust that could be measured on the Richter scale. I simply said, "I hope this never happens to them or you."

A few seconds later, I heard her call to me, "Ma'am! Ma'am! Where is your ticket? I'll take care of it for you." Well, once I'm pissed off, there's no going back. I wasn't about to beg for anyone's sympathy. Prideful, maybe. A beggar, never. "No, I don't need your help." I wanted to make her feel worse than I did. My footsteps and my words were frigid; I'm surprised my tears didn't freeze as they trickled down past the corners of my mouth.

She caught up to me when I got to my car, insisting that I give her the ticket. I was sitting in my car, crying hard now; and in public to boot. How humiliating. I couldn't even look her in the eye. She took the ticket and gave me a pass for two hours of free parking. She said, "Please, enjoy a walk on the beach." Right, enjoy myself. Sure thing, lady.

Maybe life sends us what we need in the form of bitch. If it weren't for this little altercation, I may not have surrendered to the necessary wailing fit that came over me. As I drove away, I cried harder and harder. "I'm so sorry Erik. I'm so sorry Erik." I'd manage to scream out words between the wailing. "I'm so sorry Erik. Oh my God, I'm so sorry." My voice groaned and groveled like a possessed woman. With my full blown grief out of control, I had to pull over. I wasn't able to drive as I gagged and choked on my snot, in agony over my son's agony.

That purging lasted about fifteen minutes. My vengeful pride almost kept me from using the free parking pass. But I humbled myself, accepted her apology in the form of a parking pass and drove to the dead end of Wrightsville Beach to do something for my son and myself; walk. It was my own Code Blue; the blue of sadness, sorrow and grief; the Code Blue that can only be helped by nature, ocean waves and the presence of God.

Vanity, Stars & Scars

On a Friday night, after two weeks in Rehab we took Erik on a doctor approved outing to a bar in Wilmington. Although the outing went well, it was a slap of reality in the face, at least for me and I think for Erik as well. Even so, he was gaining confidence. His dogmatic determination to be independent and free from the hospital soon prompted a round of sparring with his attending physiatrist. Erik wanted a free pass to come and go as he pleased, with no curfew. He'd been coming and going as he pleased since he was a teenager. This place of curfew and protocol was anything but his cup of tea. The physiatrist responded, "If you're feeling that good, I'd say it's time for your discharge. How about Thursday, four days from now?" Erik looked at me. I looked at the doctor, understanding that he was drawing his line of authority in the sand. When the doctor left the room, Erik asked me if I thought he was ready for discharge. "No freakin' way, Erik. No way. You're not strong enough yet. You're not healed enough yet. The incision from you spinal fusion is a mess and we have no accommodations prepared. Do you want to live with me, in a handicap hotel room?" The idea of living with me was probably enough to scare him. Erik decided to suck it up and squelch his defiance a bit longer.

Erik's Rehab team met and decided on a discharge date of June 10th, a few weeks away. And it was a good thing the discharge date was moved. It turned out Erik had a staph infection in his spinal fusion wound. I noticed seepage on his bed sheets for about five days that didn't look right so I did my own investigation. I was helping him shower one morning and applied pressure to his incision area. Puss gushed out like a volcano erupting. I could see a suture inside the hole that had formed from the volcanic eruption. It was no wonder the wound wouldn't heal. The suture wouldn't dissolve. I was furious that no one had noticed this infection building. I got testy with a nurse and Erik settled me down.

"Quiet Mom. Don't make her mad. I just want to get out of here."
He'd already ticked off this particular nurse by taping a silly note to his door that read "*Peep Show 25¢*" which she didn't appreciate and took down immediately. Erik and I both surmised that his body was rejecting the suture that didn't dissolve. He asked the neurosurgeon to remove it; perhaps our previous discussion with him regarding the shard was so heated, the request fell upon deaf ears. Or perhaps they all just thought we were bossy maniacs. Anyway, the suture remained in Erik's surgical wound, and so did the infection.

The newly diagnosed staph infection in the surgical wound was as stubborn as Erik. His back would require another debridement surgery to remove the infected tissue and cleanse the entire wound thoroughly with antibiotic. It freaked me out. I'd heard horror stories about MRSA. And there was always a whisper of that possibility lingering on the lips of Infectious Disease Specialist who visited frequently. I was very nervous about the whole thing. Were we headed back *into the woods*? The surgical wound from the debridement was left wide open and packed with a sponge that was attached to a wound vacuum, allowing it to heal slowly from the inside out. When I said "left wide open", I meant it. The wound was about nine inches long by two inches wide and very deep. They had to expose the titanium hardware to make sure it had not become infected. I watched as the first sponge was changed and the surgical wound down his back revealed it all; his spine, the rods, the screws, everything. Ugh. He didn't flinch at all during those dressing changes; the heavy doses of medications and his high tolerance to pain were working in areas where he could feel sensation. That wound vacuum would become part of Erik's permanent luggage for about two months after he left Rehab.

And now that we had a discharge date, there was a lot to do in a short period of time. It didn't seem possible. How would we manage? Where would he go? Jenny was campaigning for her home. She wanted Erik to move in with her. It wasn't an easy decision for Erik to make. To start with, we already uncovered his trust issue. And although he loved Jenny and wanted to be with her, he did not want to burden her.

To boot, he didn't want to hurt his father's feelings by leaving Wilmington and moving three hours away to Mebane where Jenny lived; it was like he was emotionally breaking up with his dad. He was also concerned about the logistics of someone being able to physically help handle him. He knew Jenny, at 4'9" tall and weighing 95 pounds, wasn't strong enough to move his 6'3", 165 pound body. Upon approval from Jenny, I offered to move in with them, just until he became independent and they were comfortable with everything.

The following entry from a prior Facebook entry might be how Erik made his decision.

Erik's Facebook

Erik Fugunt

You know right or wrong by the feeling in your chest not your head

December 20, 2010 at 12:17pm

Erik must have listened to the feeling in his chest. He decided to move to Jenny's directly out of Rehab. Once that was settled, I spent a rushed few weeks orchestrating the alterations to Jenny's house. Erik's father and friends pitched in with labor and together with a few hired contractors, Jenny's house was ready with a new ramp in the garage to access entry to the house. Erik insisted that we not make her house ugly with a ramp to the front door. We gutted and remodeled her bathroom to make it completely wheelchair accessible and rearranged furniture to make space maneuverable for Erik.

Jenny was unbelievably tolerant and benevolent. She opened her home to Erik and me, without hesitation, almost as if she had planned it this way her entire life. I can't explain it. The whole story continued to be unbelievable.

In a mad rush to prepare for his discharge, the last two weeks in Rehab went quickly. I visited Chapel Hill and arranged Erik's transfer of care to UNC Rehab Center and the appropriate physicians in that area so that Erik would not have to make a three hour trip back to Wilmington for the numerous follow ups that were scheduled. I was also able to spend a few days with Chuck. He'd flown into Raleigh for business so I met him at Jenny's house in nearby Mebane. We visited with her that evening and got to see her in her own environment. It was a much needed break and reminded me that there was life other than Erik and the hospital. It was my first time away from Erik overnight since the accident.

I was dog-tired. But this was a tired I was used to. This was a tired that came from tasking, my vice. I'd been doing a lot of inner work during the past three years; inner work using the Enneagram as a tool of spiritual and personal growth. As an Enneagram Achiever type, I'd become much more aware of how tasks and achievements were like drugs to me, an addiction. And I was in full swing. So full that it was time for a sobering moment. After my short visit with Chuck, I drove back to Wilmington for just that. And who better to serve up a sobering moment than my darling son, Erik Wolfgang.

That moment began as I accompanied Erik to the Rehab gym. He was looking for his Physical Therapist, Amber, aka Little Hitler, to repair his wheelchair. Unable to locate her, a few other physical therapists tried to assist him and decided to put him in a different wheelchair until they could fix the one he was currently using. They began to hurriedly make adjustments to a wheelchair that Erik hated in order to make him use it. Nuh uh! Not going to happen!

Erik defiantly rolled himself out of there like a bat out of hell leaving fumes of fury and frustration trailing as he bellowed, "Like hell you'll put me in that chair!"

I stood frozen. My son had acted disrespectful to these ladies. The shock and disdain on their faces clearly indicated their disapproval of his behavior. And wasn't I responsible for my son's behavior? I was horrified. To get me off the bad parenting hook, I apologized to the ladies and remarked arrogantly in my defense, "Can you tell he grew up with his father?" How lame of me.

I caught up with Erik in the elevator and followed him back to his room where the real lesson began. I started to scold him, reprimanding him for his disrespectful behavior. His face was red and ready to explode with anger and tears. I continued to scold him. Amber, his preferred therapist, entered the room in the midst of this, apologizing to Erik. I guess she had promised to fix his chair for him. She felt horrible that he couldn't find her so she offered to fix it right now. Well, Miss High and Mighty Mama (me) said to her, "Amber, don't you reward his bad behavior!"

With that, Erik busted into tears and it's a wonder he didn't bust into me. I was taken back. Something had shifted at that moment. I said, "Amber, I think we need some *mother and son* time." She nodded her head in agreement with an understanding smile and left us alone.

"Erik, honey I'm sorry. I can't even begin to imagine how frustrated and angry you must be. I'm so sorry. I was just embarrassed with how you spoke to those ladies downstairs."

Erik lifted his head to look at me; his eyes were red from tears, frustration and anger. "Embarrassed," he scoffed. "So I'm an embarrassment to you." He spun away from me like a top and wheeled to the bathroom. My lesson was sinking in at warp speed.

I gasped in horror at my own self. How could I be so vain, so caught up in what was appropriate or what other people thought of me?

I was disgusted with myself and ashamed that I'd made my own son feel like an embarrassment. I gathered myself with calm intention as humiliation was flooding my soul. Crying, I walked to the bathroom where I found Erik hanging over the sink, sobbing his heart out.

I stood behind him and fumbled words out of my mouth between my own sobs, "Erik, YOU are not an embarrassment. You could never be an embarrassment to me. I am so proud of you. You're my pride and joy. Everything you've gone through, what you've endured, you're amazing. I was embarrassed with your behavior because I felt it reflected my mothering skills. That's my problem, not yours. That's my deficiency, not yours. The hell with my mothering skills and the hell with what other people think of me. *I love you* Erik and I'm proud of you. You will never be an embarrassment. I'm so sorry."

As I cried, I placed my hands over my mouth as if it might somehow keep those ugly, hurtful things I'd already said from escaping my lips ever again or somehow take them back. We sat silently in the bathroom for what seemed like forever, until Jason, Erik's friend stopped for a visit and interrupted the silence. His timely appearance was like a ringing bell that indicated class and this lesson had ended. I quietly excused myself.

Although I don't condone disrespectful behavior, I also don't condone my vanity. The next day, we practiced a transfer into my car and I took him for a slow ride in my car through the hospital parking lot. We talked about what happened the day before. I told him that we were different for good reason; so we could learn from each other. I told him I'd learned a lot from him and that learning would never end. I also suggested that just maybe, he could learn something from me too.

At day's end, I was thankful for a son who was bold enough to stand up to me, patient enough to tolerate me and forgiving enough to love me despite my vanity and workaholic nature.

Like clockwork, following that emotional valley and recovery, Superman made his routine visit. To our surprise, he asked us to participate in the Leadership Development Institute. Tom wanted us to share our story with the leadership of the hospital since Erik had been through every facet of their institution. From EMS to Rehab, from Hospitality House to Kona Café, we'd been touched by someone in every single department of that hospital.

We gave Tom a list of people that had made the biggest impact on us, respectively. He laughed and said the list was too long, he'd have to close the hospital to get them all there, but he'd see what he could do. The event was scheduled for June 9th, the day before Erik's discharge. Neither Erik nor I had a written speech prepared. We figured we'd just go by the seat of our pants, the best way to fly.

Meanwhile, Erik had one more special visitor before he was discharged. It suddenly hit me that a visit from this guy might do a world of good for Erik so I got his phone number from Erik's friend, Jason, and gave him a call. No answer, so I left a message. I'd never met this man but knew it was someone very special from what Erik had shared with me. Within a few minutes, he returned my call. He was on his way, just like that, to the hospital to see Erik. It was a special visit; a very special visit.

The following passage from Facebook that Erik wrote after meeting this man five months prior, explains it all.

Erik's Facebook

Something happened to me today that is one of the rarest gifts that could ever be given. I had a life changing experience. I met a man named Elmer Hayes. The gentleman in his early sixties was educated, strong-willed and from the first moment he spoke I knew there was something different about him apart from the fact that he was almost completely deaf from birth. A German native, he moved to the USA in his early teens.

He faced challenges and obstacles I could only imagine and yet he had a love and passion for life that I have only seen in a handful of people. As we talked and I asked questions about his wife, children, house, motorcycles, woodworking and numerous pictures of sailboats on the wall, he opened his life to me in the most true and honest way he possibly could. As fate would have it, he was a mariner, a man who lived for over seven years along with his wife aboard a sailboat. The couple lived and played on this vessel for a few years before they had children. While raising a son and daughter they began to sail the oceans with young ones on board. They went all over the Atlantic and some of the Pacific oceans together as a family.

While he told me stories of adventure, relaxation, bonding, passion and love, snickering at his – as he called "boring neighbors" – it hit me this was a man that had the same beliefs, passions and love for life that I have always cherished and lived by. As his stories went on about the people he had met, his adventures and romance, my mind became as clear as the crystal waters in the lagoon he described in such detail that it brought tears to my eyes. After he realized how moved I was by their life he stopped and looked at me with a smile and said, "What are you waiting for?" I smiled back and replied, "A life changing moment."

A life changing moment. Erik knew his moment with Elmer Hayes was life changing, yet a moment soon to follow on April 14, 2010 would be the most monumental life changing moment my son would ever know. If Erik meeting Elmer a few months ago was a coincidence, then I have to believe Albert Einstein when he quoted, **"Coincidence is God's way of remaining anonymous."** Elmer brought his wife and they visited with Erik for a long time. It was great, to meet them personally and to watch them interact with my son.

The day of the Leadership Development Institute event came quickly. Erik took his good old time getting ready that morning, running late, as usual. That's one thing that had not changed a bit; his notorious lollygagging. I seriously think he likes people waiting for him. Perhaps it makes for a more grandiose entrance and gives him control. Anyway, a transport van picked Erik up at the hospital. He'd been out of Rehab on day passes before, in which he'd struggle to transfer himself from his wheelchair into a car. Once in the car, his biggest challenge was his balance but for the most part he would ride like a normal passenger. This time, he was wheeled in the back of a large transport van, remained seated in his wheelchair and was strapped down like cargo.

Noa, his Occupational Therapist and I rode with him in the van and kept an eye on him. We noticed that he got a little freaked out. He didn't like it at all. It was hard enough for him to be a passenger with someone else at the wheel and in control but in that situation he always felt like he could at least grab the wheel if he needed to make a heroic maneuver to avoid a crash. And actually, he'd done that before with a friend in Maryland, to avoid a head on collision and may have saved both their lives. But now, strapped in the back of a van like cargo, he was completely vulnerable. The look of untrusting terror was in his eyes.

Then I remembered reading about Christopher Reeves. He had the same reaction when he first experienced himself being hauled around like cargo. Luckily the venue for the Leadership Development Institute was not far away.

Upon our arrival, Tom guided us to a room filled with most of the health care workers that we'd requested to be there. He apologized for not having the complete list but joked that he'd have to close the hospital to get them all there. In that back room, Tom's assistant, Meri played a power point presentation that she created for the presentation. She'd gathered photographs that I'd taken with my cell phone during the last eight weeks, along with a few photos that the hospital photographer had taken and used music from *Footprints in the Sand* by Leona Lewis to accompany the photographs and subtitles, telling Erik's gripping story with overwhelming emotional impact.

As our little group previewed it, the only sounds that could be heard above the music of the power point were that of sniffling and nose-blowing. The lyrics were absolutely perfect...

You walked with me, footprints in the sand,
and helped me understand where I'm going.

You walked with me, when I was all alone,
with so much unknown along the way – and I heard you say,

I promise you, I'm always there,
when your heart is filled with sadness and despair.

I'll carry you, when you need a friend -
you'll find my footprints in the sand.

We all tried to collect ourselves to make an entrance on the stage. Superman Tom prefaced our entrance with the story of how he'd met Erik in the ICU, just eight weeks ago. Tom summarized that conversation and conveyed how impressed he was with Erik's ability to communicate in spite of the tracheotomy and even more impressed that Erik managed to shake his hand and thank him for stopping by. But what really touched the heart of Superman was something my son told him a few weeks after they first met. Erik told him that he never realized how many people really loved him until this happened. That was a huge take away for Tom. He shared with the audience that none of us really ever know the difference we make in one another's lives and encouraged everyone to take a moment to think about that.

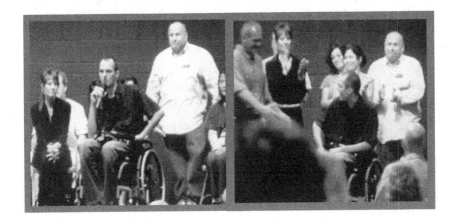

Erik's presentation

That was our cue to take the stage. Along with the entourage of Erik's health care workers that we had asked to be with us, we all made our way to seats on the stage. As we did, Meri's power point was playing, larger than life, on various big screens throughout the auditorium for the attendees to view.

There were about three hundred hospital personnel present; even the big wigs, who were seated right in front of us. The music and message was heart wrenchingly powerful for everyone involved. Each and every person could relate in some way or another to a time of their life that was bleak; a time that that reminded them about the footprints in their own sand. And now they were being shown that they were part of someone else's sandy beach. Each one of them had made a footprint in our sand, a mark in our lives. Yes, those footprints would erode in time, as the days of our lives, like water, would erase the visible imprint. But the invisible imprint would never be erased. It was part of our lives now. It was stored in our hearts and our purpose there that day was to tell them.

Meri's presentation flawlessly revealed the human interest side of Erik's story. It delivered a powerful and succinct message to the attendees of the conference; that every employee in the hospital, from the Janitor to the President, from Nurse Assistant to Neurosurgeon, from Cashier to Cook, from the Hospitality House Host to the Shuttle Bus Driver, has the power to make a difference in a patient's life. We passed out a lot of Kleenex, even at the onset. That power point hit the audience early with an emotional impact and set the stage for my son to deliver his own magic. And it was priceless.

The way Erik conducted himself in front of that group was something I'd never seen; unrehearsed words flowing with heartache and humor. His opening remarks went like this, "I understand that this is a pretty big deal and that you're the head honchos – the ones I used to call nerds in high school. Turns out I'm sorry I put that sign on your back! Ya know?" The audience roared with laughter. He continued. "They brought me here today to pretty much – well, I was told that I'm supposed to inspire you guys." There was a long unrehearsed pause which created even more suspense. "Well I'm here –" and he started to sob. Applause broke loose. When it ceased, he finished, "– and uh, it's kinda – a big deal for me."

Tom, Superman, was standing close by and handed him a tissue. Erik wiped the tears from his face, let out a deep sigh and apologized for becoming emotional. "Thanks, Tom." He regained his composure with the perfectly timed witty response to the crowd. "Superman. I told him to check his cape at the door." He elicited another hearty dose of laughter from everyone! I remember sitting there behind him, completely awestruck. I was thinking, "Who is this kid? He's a natural; so poised with laughter and tears in front of hundreds of people."

He continued. "But honestly, I never really expected to survive through this kind of injury. I always knew it was a possibility that I would be hurt. Those are the risks we take. But I think living through it has been harder than if I would've let go. So there's got to be a reason. And uh, hopefully, coming in front of you guys today and letting you know that I'm appreciative – " Erik's voice faded again as he began to cry. The crowd began to applaud him again. He wiped his nose and quickly finished his thought, "– that might be some of the reason."

To my knowledge, Erik had never addressed a large audience before. Yet, he commanded that crowd with genuine emotion, candid humor and sincerity; all delivered with piercing communication skills. No one would have guessed that he had a huge open wound down his back from the recent debridement or that he was attached to a wound vacuum; we tucked it underneath the wheelchair using huge elastic exercise bands. I have to give some credit to the drugs but honestly, he engaged that audience like a professional motivational speaker. I was so very proud of my son.

The hospital staff that was involved in Erik's care was on stage with us. Each of them had a few moments to share a story and talk with Erik in front of the audience. Bill, the respiratory hero from the Trauma Team was the first to begin. He gave the audience a quick summary of Erik's arrival, how they frantically fought for his life and literally ran down the hallway with their hands in his chest to look for the first available operating room.

Bill continued and shared how he had worked on two other motorcycle accident patients that week and that they didn't make it. Bringing his tissue to his eyes and referring to Erik's survival, he said, "So I really needed his victory." The emotion he displayed was incredible. I was so touched by it. Everyone was. And it set the stage for the rest of the health care workers to share their own very personal story of their time with Erik.

Aaron, his ICU Nurse, spilled the beans about how it was his first tour of duty in ICU when Erik has arrived. By far, Erik was the worst patient he'd ever seen. But he followed protocol and didn't expose his rookie status, encouraging Erik all along that he was going to be just fine. Erik looked at him and just shook his head, saying "Aw man, you're kidding! You did a good job of pulling it off. Maybe there's a career in acting someday for you?"

ICU Nurse Nikki shared a personal story about how Erik's feisty personality inspired her to keep fighting in difficult time of her own life; and ICU Nurse Louise read a poem to Erik about the hummingbird and how the special essence of that little creature reminded her of the special relationship that formed between all of us as we cared for him together in ICU. Manley, the transporter, conveyed his affection towards Erik by giving him a NASCAR shirt, number 24. He cried too, as he shared how his mother, even though deceased, could send love to him through another woman, by watching me care for my son. Ben, the paramedic, spoke so softly, not only moved emotionally by Erik's survival but humbly appreciative of being included in the aftermath of his efforts. Every health care worker on that stage spoke. Even the ones that had previously declined speaking on stage now had found the courage to share their respective stories.

I also had the opportunity to share my experiences, throughout the eight week ordeal, conveying my thanks to the hospital for their respectfulness of the different modalities of medicine that I had practiced throughout Erik's stay.

I thanked Doctor Mindy Merritt who couldn't make it and said I wanted her to know how proud her father was of her, for saving my son's life. I thanked Louise for watching over Erik in ICU, physically and spiritually, because I didn't know if he would be alive by the time I arrived. I summarized with, "So, what's the saying? To love another is to see the face of God. Well, I've seen a lot of God. I see a lot of God in all your faces." I reached to affectionately rub Erik's head and finished, "My favorite just happens to be right here, right now. Thank you for keeping him with us." I cried, kissed his forehead and made my way back to my seat.

Erik took the microphone one last time. After chiding me about being an emotional wreck and thanking everyone again, his final message revealed his true nature. He spoke reverently and tearfully this time, saying, "The most meaningful impact was not really the care towards me. It was the care towards the ones I love." His voice began to quiver with emotion. "The doors were open. My father and mother were allowed to come and see me anytime they wanted. My girlfriend was allowed to stay with me. Those were the things that mean way more than any surgery could ever repair. So thank you, for keeping the doors open. That's it." And that was it. A presentation scheduled for thirty minutes took sixty minutes and every precious minute was perfect.

That auditorium was transformed into a glowing safe haven of loving gratitude in which no one could hold back their heart's language. There was a complete representation of every hospital department on that stage and we'd seen them all. Until that time, each of them only knew their little piece of the story. After everyone had shared their personal anecdotes, a beautiful mosaic of the bigger picture was created. A new appreciation for the entire story was revealed with a lengthy standing ovation.

Other than Erik's very small and simple graduation dinner from American Motorcycle Institute, there were no other marked events in his life for me to attend. Indeed, this was a shining star moment. Erik was a star, not a movie star, a real life star.

Who better to know a star when he met one, than a man that flies among them? Superman, Tom VP. I guess that's why he asked Erik to speak. He saw into the heart of Erik. Why, of course he did. Superman has x-ray vision.

The next evening Thursday, June 10th at 7:45 in the evening, Erik was finally discharged from New Hanover Regional Rehab Hospital, just eight weeks after his crash. I say "just eight weeks" now. But it was a lifetime then. That morning, I drove to the scene of his accident for the first time. I parked my car and got out to walk around. It was void. I had no feeling at all; as if it didn't even happen. The tree of impact was gone; his dad had taken care of that. Everything was nicely landscaped and looked peaceful. I drove away and said a quiet farewell to Erik's old legs. I could almost see them floating toward Heaven.

On the day of his discharge, Erik had some very special visitors with very special messages: Superman, of course, with the proverbial "If you ever need *anything,* just call me" – Don Knowles, the gentlemen that lived by the crash site spoke with Erik and assured him that God had a plan for his life, no matter what it seemed liked now, God would show him the way – Marilyn, his massage therapist brought a lovely table trivet inscribed with a bible verse.

"For I know the plans I have for you, to give you hope and a future."
Jeremiah 29:11

Bill, the Respiratory Therapist that worked on Erik in the ER, spoke ever so tenderly with Erik and asked him to remember the intimacies of life that are so precious and so overlooked, like the touch of woman and the love of a heart. David, the hospital writer, made a last minute appearance as well. He was trying to facilitate an interview with Erik by the local TV station before we left for Mebane. It didn't pan out. The reporter was called to cover another breaking news story. Stardom was over. Life at New Hanover Regional Medical Center and Rehabilitation Hospital was over, finally.

Bill, the trauma team respiratory hero with Erik

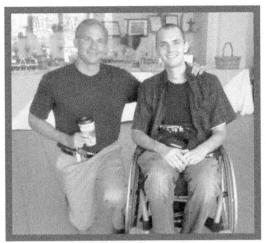

after the LDI presentation

Dark storm clouds were moving in. It was a fitting ending as I loaded the last bit of Erik's stuff into my already over packed car. I parked curbside and left the passenger door open to welcome Erik, then went back inside to wheel him out. It was surreal, such an unassuming exit. No nurses, no attendees, no anybody, just Erik and me and a quick goodbye from the right-hand man, Joe. By the time I got him wheeled outside, the threatening storm clouds had broken loose. Rain was slamming down. The sky was dark and ominous with thunder and lightning. As I struggled to get Erik into the car, a man jumped out of his truck and held an umbrella over us the best he could. His gesture was kind and appreciated, but ineffective. We were soaking wet. I was nervous but figured if anything went wrong during our three hour journey to Jenny's house in Mebane, I'd just call 911 or rush to the nearest Emergency Room. Erik didn't seem scared at all, just worried, about his future, all the obstacles and all the unknowns.

As we drove off into that storm, Erik asked me, "Mom, what do you think is going to happen to me?"

His voice was as foreboding as the dark stormy sky.

"I don't know, Erik." I paused a few seconds. "I believe you will walk again, but I don't know how."

"You just believe that because you hope that," he said quietly with realism laced in his tone.

"Maybe," I said "I don't know. But you asked me what I thought would happen to you. I believe you will walk again. I don't know how – on your own, with braces, mechanically, somehow. I believe you will walk again. I can't explain it. I just believe it."

It was a long ominous ride that night to Mebane, storms, detours and all. So if we were finally *out of the woods*, where in hell were we now? I was anxious. I hoped that Erik couldn't tell. I'd been living by means of my credit card for two months. For the first time in my life, I'd asked my parents for financial help. And I begged my credit card company for a hefty increase in credit. Friends and family had sent money too. But since I always prided myself in running a pretty tight ship, I was stunned that my expenses were well over ten thousand dollars already. Even so, there was no way I was willing to wait for public assistance from Independent Living to install a ramp or bathroom. That could take months. And I was hell bound on keeping Erik full of vitamins, supplements and the freshest foods and juices. He was open to the idea of having acupuncture treatments at Chapel Hill and massage treatments at home. So I just kept plowing ahead. Thank God for the Wilmington Hospitality House and their lodging accommodations or my overall debt of sixteen thousand would have been much higher. So far I'd been able to fly by the seat of my pants and make it. I just needed to hang on through the summer. I convinced myself that I could do it and regroup when I got back to Pennsylvania.

The long drive was nice in some ways. We talked about a lot of things, without having to make direct eye contact. It's easier that way somehow, to say things you wouldn't normally say. As mechanically-minded as Erik is, he is equally philosophical. We talked about the dynamics of his relationship with Jenny and how special she was. We brainstormed about an invention; a device that would make his bowel program faster and cleaner.

At one point, I even had him take the wheel from the passenger seat and he drove for a while. And the further from Wilmington we got, the more the storm eased up. We were about half an hour away from Jenny's when a detour sign took us out of our way. Oh boy, just what I needed; a detour on a dark stormy night, in a strange land, with a newly paralyzed son in the passenger seat and most of his belongings stuffed in my back seat and trunk. I was looking to the sky, waiting for it to clear, hoping to spot a star somewhere out there, to wish upon; but there were no stars to be found, not that night. My star was not in the sky. It was in the heart of an amazing young lady named Jenny. We finally arrived at her home at 11 o'clock that night; vanity, stars, and scars. For the first time in eight weeks, Erik felt safe at home and he fell asleep in a real bed with Jenny by his side. I took a deep breath and made my way to the spare bedroom that we'd set up with an air mattress. I too, finally slept, for real.

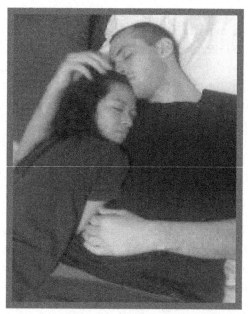

Jenny and Erik, his first night home

Going Home

You'd think it would have been awkward, moving into someone else's home; someone who was a complete stranger just eight weeks ago. Jenny made it anything but awkward. I tended to Erik like a mama bear and became Hazel, just like the famous maid from an old television sitcom. Erik's visiting nurse, Vickie was fantastic. She was perfect, a good old-fashioned nurse, not just collecting a paycheck. She was highly skilled and loaded with common sense, compassion and grit. We all loved her. I knew Erik would receive superb care under her watch.

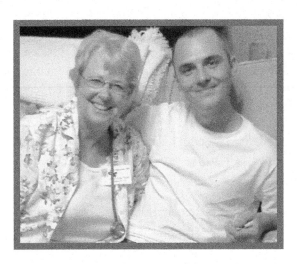

Nurse Vickie and Erik
moments before I left for home

Before I could leave them to their own devices and return to Pennsylvania, I had an agenda to accomplish and Erik had a few items of his own on that agenda. Number one – detox. A week after he got home, he quit taking all his meds, cold turkey, with no doctor's supervision.

One morning as he lay in bed, he looked up at me and said, "I'm tired of feeling like shit. No more pain meds or pills." He ripped the patch of Torodal off his upper arm. He'd been taking approximately twenty Oxycodone tablets a day and refused to take any more. I had no idea what was about to happen; an old fashioned honest to goodness detoxification. Those next four days were horrendous. He was so sick. We dragged him to the shower and dragged the bed linens to the back yard; both needed a good hosing down. It was such a mess. I won't even describe it in detail. I will tell you that once we got him cleaned up, he lived in the shower for four days.

The mad rush to make Jenny's bathroom handicap accessible really paid off, or we would have had an even bigger mess on our hands. He would sit in that shower with hot water trickling over him for hours. It was the only thing that provided him with some relief. Then we'd put him in bed for about an hour until he couldn't tolerate the nausea and the feeling of worms crawling out of his body. Then we'd drag him back to the shower again. Four days of that, four days of another hellish scene, and then it was over, just like that.

We had a scheduled visit with his new doctors at UNC in Chapel Hill a few days after the whole horrible ordeal. They said, "Erik we need to start weaning you off the pain meds."

"Already done, I'm not taking anything. Stopped, cold turkey, last week." Erik looked them right in the eye. His attitude was growing ever more defiant. His anger with his condition was building. They looked at me in disbelief. I just raised my eyebrows and shrugged my shoulders.

"He's tough," I said. The doctor just shook their heads. Erik told them that massage, chiropractic care and acupuncture were now the most effective treatments for his pain relief. At the time, I really had no idea how dangerous it was for him to stop taking the pain meds cold turkey. What's the saying? What you don't know won't hurt you. This time, it could have. We got lucky, again. It was definitely the hardest physiological part of the transition to being home.

The hardest emotional part of the transition was getting a second opinion from the neurosurgeon in Chapel Hill regarding the shattered T9 vertebra. Erik and I had still been holding on to the hope that someone else would remove the shard of bone and open the pathway of the spinal column. That was a negative, regarding the removal of the shard *and* Erik's state of mind. When the second opinion concurred with his current surgery, Erik was beyond angry. He wheeled through the hallways of UNC like a maniac; wheelchair road rage. He was ready to check out and I don't mean check out of the hospital. I'm talking the big "check out". We were waiting for the valet in front of UNC when Erik phoned his "check out" buddy, calling in the favor.

I couldn't hear their conversation. I didn't need to. I could feel what was going on. When we got home, he told me to get some life insurance on him. I yelled at him, telling him I didn't want to hear that crap. I wasn't going to get life insurance on him. I was betting on him to live – not die. And besides, who was going to sell me life insurance when the suicide rate for paraplegics is so high? I didn't pull any punches. And I didn't fight this hard for him to give up now. I left the house to cool off and when I returned, I semi-apologized. I acknowledged that if I were in his position, I'd probably feel the same way. And if he were in my position, he'd be shouting the same things I did. He said, "I know Mom. You're just fighting for your son's life. And you're doing a good job." Darn him. As quickly as he can make me mad, he can melt me into a puddle of goo.

While I stayed with Jenny and Erik, I slept on an air mattress in her spare bedroom. I must say it was paradise compared to the hospital days. Waking up in a real home, the same home that Jenny and my son now occupied was somewhat comforting. Things were beginning to feel like they might be almost normal – someday. Erik would call me from his cell phone during the night or early morning, when he needed assistance. I was getting some decent sleep but craved even more. One morning, shortly after I awoke I had a sudden vision in my mind of the woman who wouldn't meet with us; the eyewitness who said she'd visit but then never showed up. I couldn't get her out of my mind. As I showered, brushed my teeth and dried my hair, I couldn't help but review my conversations and voice messages with her. My mind began to whirr. Why didn't she visit us? What is she hiding?

Earlier that week, Erik told me that he'd experienced a few flashbacks of a dark colored SUV or minivan type vehicle and then remembered skidding backwards on his bottom saying, "Oh f – – k." I couldn't help but wonder. Was the eyewitness that wouldn't meet with us driving a vehicle that fit that description?

Suspicion replaced my sympathy for her. I couldn't quit thinking about it. And the longer I thought about it, the more suspicious I became. She said she saw his bike begin to wobble and then watched him crash in her rear view mirror. Did the spill initiate the wobbling? Did he wobble into her as they were approaching the curve coming towards each other? Is that why his left hand was broken? Did it hit her mirror? Was she involved in the accident? Did she run him off the road? Why did she keep driving and call her daughter instead of calling 911 first? My heart began to race. By now, almost two months had passed since the accident. But something wasn't right. I felt it, in my gut. So I called the State Police in Wilmington, the same troopers that I had visited shortly after the accident to show them my pictures of the spill on the road. I explained my "gut" feeling. Their response was respectfully curt. "Even if she did run him off the road, she wouldn't admit it." Now, I know the police have a difficult job. I know that kids on bikes speed. I know the love-hate relationship that exists between law enforcement and crotch rockets. I know the police report stated that the accident was due to speeding. I know that many times, speed kills. And I know my son. I know he speeds. And I know his riding abilities. Was it really just speed that caused the accident? I persisted. The officer agreed to visit the woman to ask for a statement and reminded me that she was not obligated to do so.

I was appalled. How could she be excused from having to provide an official statement when she was the only eyewitness? I was livid. I'm not sure if it was a delayed need for blame or if it was a moment of clarity. Either way, I wanted an official statement from the woman. The only person that had any insight into the accident hadn't even been interviewed at the time. I was pissed and sassy with the officer who said he'd get back with me after he made a visit to her. I struggled emotionally that day, wondering if I should tell Erik that I made the phone call to the police. I decided to hold my tongue and wait to see how the officer replied.

It didn't take long for the officer to get back to me. The woman agreed to provide a short statement. "She saw Erik at the bend. His bike began to wobble. He looked behind him. He lost control and hit a tree." She explained to the officer that she never met with us because she was having nightmares about it and her husband told her not to meet with us. It was too traumatic.

Really? Too traumatic? How about that? I guess what Erik had been through wasn't traumatic. Oh. I was seething. I questioned the officer regarding the possibilities. I told him that I smelled a rat; that something wasn't right. The officer reminded me that they are professionals and that I would just have to accept the fact that they did their job; accept the fact that speeding was the cause of the accident. I thanked him for his time and told him that although it wouldn't change anything, he would just have to accept that fact that I smelled a rat.

I remember a wise old lawyer telling me years ago, that if you smell a rat – there's usually a rat. The woman's statement actually supported Ron's theory that the spill across the road caused the bike to wobble. This woman said that Erik turned to look behind him. An experienced rider doesn't do that, unless there is darn good reason. Maybe he looked back to see what he'd just rode through. Maybe the spill caused the bike to wobble. But it didn't matter now. None of our theories mattered. The authorities could not be persuaded to investigate further. It was good enough for them, but not me.

Later that afternoon, after much lamenting I told Erik about my phone call to the Wilmington State Police and their response. Erik actually consoled me with his insightful words, "It doesn't change anything Mom. Even if someone is liable, it would be nice to hear that they were sorry, but nothing changes the fact that I'm paralyzed. And if it doesn't change that, it doesn't really matter." His wisdom and discernment far surpassed mine at that point. And his forgiving nature was still intact.

The six weeks that I stayed with him and Jenny were the most rewarding six weeks I'd ever known with my son. I have so many good memories that equalize the sad ones. Like the time I dragged him against his gloom and doom outlook, to Lowes to look for a part to complete the **Paraflush™**, a great apparatus that he invented for a quick and clean bowel program. I'd been to Lowes almost daily, rigging up odds and ends to make this thing work, but we were having some mechanical snags. And he was *sure* there was nothing at Lowes that would work. He gave me such an attitude. I literally dragged him to that store. Lowes and behold, he found it, a part that would work, for now. I'd seen it earlier and completely dismissed it. Not eagle eye Erik. He nabbed it up. Back home in the bathroom, he connected it and it worked! There was still room for improvement with his design but he was definitely in business with a device that provided for a clean and easy bowel program. Hot Diggity Dog!

"Really, I ought to kick your butt!" I grinned like a Cheshire cat and began to mock his words like a whiney little school kid, "They won't have anything. I'm not going to Lowes; they won't have nothin' that works. Pout. Pout. Poor me." I was tired of him acting like a gimp and feeling sorry for himself. He was anything but a gimp. So I teased him relentlessly.

He was having a great laugh. "Go ahead, kick my butt! I can't feel it anyway!" What a smart ass.

Now I'm laughing, "I'll just kick your head then. Don't think I can't reach it!" I lifted my leg, pretending to kick him in the noggin, all in fun of course. With that he took the sprayer from the **Paraflush**™ and soaked me from head to toe. That little shit. No pun intended! We had a hardy laugh in the bathroom that night; a real laugh. It felt so good. When we finished the water battle, I firmly reminded him, "See? Never give up, ever."

We had another "*Optimistic versus Pessimistic*" event occur at UNC Hospital. Erik had transferred from the car to his wheelchair at valet parking, wheeled through the valet parking area, along a sidewalk, across a street, into the hospital and through crowded hallways onto an elevator, then into a 2nd floor receptionist office. He was registering for an out-patient procedure to remove the vena cava filter that had been inserted while he was in ICU to help prevent blood clots from reaching his heart and lungs. The registrar asked for his medical card. Reaching into his lap for his wallet, his face turned white. His wallet was gone. We raced to retrace our steps. "We'll find it." I assured him. "Someone will turn it in."

"Are you kidding me?" he snarled. "I had four hundred dollars in there." The money was from a benefit that his friends had held in Wilmington before he was discharged from the hospital and it was his life savings at this point. "No one's going to turn it in! Don't be crazy. It's gone."

I went to the main desk. He rolled to the parking valet who was standing at the front door. Bingo, the parking valet had found it, given it to a security guard and it was back in Erik's lap within five minutes, not a dollar missing. I loved it when my Pollyanna attitude defeated his Darth Vader gloom and doom. And when it worked to his favor, he liked it too.

One evening, close to the time I would be leaving, Jenny wanted to go out and meet some friends in Chapel Hill. It was late and Erik was tired. He didn't want to go but he didn't want his girlfriend going without him. I said, "Erik, you don't have to go. You don't have to sacrifice yourself. If you don't feel good, don't go. Jenny will be fine. Anyway, where's this martyr coming from. You never sacrifice yourself for me." I was being sarcastic and had no idea what impact that statement would have on him.

He looked straight into my soul with those weapons of his that I call eyes and said with stabbing force, "*Oh yes. I have.*" There was a chilling silence that followed. I instinctively understood where he was coming from. I felt that remark coming from a deep place, from the little boy that grew up quick and tended to some very difficult issues when I divorced his father. During that time he sacrificed; he somehow protected his mama while staying loyal and dedicated to his daddy. I nodded my head quietly, "I understand." He went out with Jenny that night. I went to bed and slept so well that I never heard them come in. Funny, you'd think I'd worry more about him more because of his condition, still healing from massive injuries, let alone paralysis. But I felt safety around him. He was used to living on wheels. Now his wheels just didn't go so fast, they were manually powered. Maybe that's why I could sleep so well.

We'd go shopping, all three of us together. He'd set Jenny on his lap and roll through the stores. I loved watching them together and watching their confidence grow. By the Fourth of July, we were all ready for a break. I flew home to celebrate the holiday with Chuck, whose father's birthday was on the Fourth of July, just like Erik's. Jenny drove Erik to Wilmington, where they would celebrate his birthday with family and friends.

chapter 14 | going home

They also met a reporter and Doctor Mindy, Erik's ER angel, for an inspiring human interest story that aired on the local news station, about a young man celebrating a birthday that no one expected him to see.

Jenny didn't miss any work. She adapted to the situation and became comfortable with Erik's condition very quickly. He convinced her to take him swimming, against doctor's orders. Seems they're both a bit rebellious. She liked to stay on the go. And she dragged him everywhere she wanted to go. It was good for him; really good for him. He had an episode on the couch one night and she ran to get me out of bed. He was faint and holding his chest. I thought he was passing a blood clot or having a heart attack. I was ready to call 911 but Erik said no. I thought to myself, "You mean to tell me we got him this far and he's going to die now?" Jenny had already looked online to see what to do. She gave him water and made him lie flat. Then we stayed with him until it passed and he felt okay again. You learn a lot about paraplegics and what happens to their bodies, when you have to. Jenny was quick, highly intelligent and feisty enough to handle Erik. It gave me such peace of mind.

There was only one more item on my agenda to ensure Erik's independence – hand controls for his car. I knew that driving would be the last major component for him to gain complete independence. The Independent Living Agency would help pay for hand controls, but again, I wasn't willing to wait for the estimated three to six months and muddle through their red tape. It was important for Erik's mental state to get him functioning independently, the sooner the better.

The first step was to have an official examiner come to the house and have Erik actually drive a car which was equipped with hand controls. I was so excited! It was a milestone of independence for both of us. Erik transferred from his wheelchair into the driver's seat of the inspector's car. His transfers were weak but he did pretty well considering that his left shoulder was still jacked up. Then off they went. He was on his own – and driving! Twenty minutes later, they returned. Erik passed, of course, with flying colors. No surprise there. We had car controls installed in Erik's car at the first appointment available. After a few naps in the waiting area for an all-day installation, Erik got in the driver's seat. The installer said to me, "Are you sure you want him to drive home? Paraplegics usually have someone else drive them home and then practice awhile before they go any distance. You have an hour drive, at least, through the city of Raleigh and this is his first time." Obviously, they didn't know Erik.

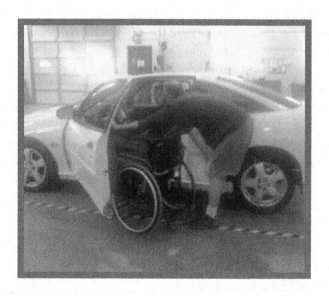

Erik with the tech that installed his hand controls

I sat in the passenger seat, looked over at Erik and asked the question to prove my point to the installer. "Can you drive home?"

"Yep." he answered. And that was that. We were off. Erik would have said yes, no matter what. He couldn't take one more minute of me driving him around or driving him crazy with my mothering.

The times in the hospital when he wanted me with him constantly were long gone. It was quite evident my purpose here was complete and it was time for me to go.

The next day, I accompanied him as he drove himself to the chiropractor. The following day I accompanied him as he drove himself to the outpatient Rehab Center, another successful jaunt that proved his capabilities to me. He could shit, shower, shave, dress and drive himself. He met the criteria of independent living according to my book. It was my last day with Erik, so his physical therapist took a photo of us together. Erik was doing great. His rehabilitation was far from complete but I was satisfied with his independence. Mission accomplished. It was time to head home, finally.

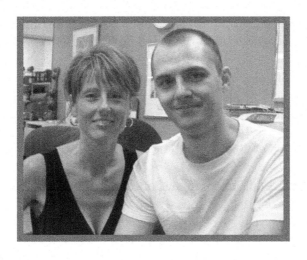

Me with Erik at ARMC Rehab the day before I left

As dramatically as this whole thing started, it ended quite mundane; funny how life works that way. It was a series of events, ones that I didn't think I could live through and ones I didn't think Erik would live through. We both did. And now it was time for him to continue his journey without me. He had his own life to live and it was to be shared with Jenny, not me.

My work here was done. I know they were appreciative of my help but I'm sure they were very happy to see me go. I was happy to see me go; and so very proud of them both.

I purposely waited to leave until Jenny was at work and Nurse Vicki was visiting with Erik. I knew it would be easier to say a casual goodbye that way. With a quick genuine hug, kiss and "love ya", I walked out the door with a smile. The following year would bring plenty of time to cry the deep tears of grief. But not now, they weren't necessary. Right now, all was well.

By now, I was quite thin, but in good physical shape overall, with not a bit of trouble from my thyroid. I'd *spoken* and *lived* my truth like never before. I'd kept a steady regiment of supplements and ate healthy. I felt good as gold. I walked a few miles every day while I stayed at Jenny's house, down and back the country road. Before I left, there was a turtle crossing the road where I walked. I carefully picked him up and moved him to the edge of the road to prevent his untimely death. That turtle spoke to me the very words God wanted me to hear. "It's time to slow down now. He will find his own way, slow and steady."

I left North Carolina on Wednesday, July 21, 2010, exactly fourteen weeks from the day I arrived; the day of Erik's accident, April 14, 2010. Those weeks were the most profound of my entire life. Never before had I been so fulfilled. Never before had I known such valleys or peaks. Never before had I known my son so well, or what it meant to love him so deeply. Never before had I been so healed. My life wasn't better or worse than before Erik's accident. It was just different. Different in ways that written words can't touch. It's sadder; yet richer somehow. Even though I still ache for my son and still weep for his loss; I also feel a peace and acceptance. I feel grace. And even though I still nag him and maybe spoil him, he still pisses me off and I tear into him with a lecture. But after I settle down, I lay my head on his lap and tell him how much I love him. And he says, "I know Mama. I love you, too." Maybe life wasn't that much different after all. Maybe we just shared a walk through hell – together.

Writing the story of this walk through hell answered a lot of questions for me. Why are we here on earth? To suffer? To learn? To love? We're here to live, plain and simple; to embrace the experience of life in a human body. And life in a human body includes all of it; the good, the bad, the ugly – even dying. Some questions aren't answerable in the language we're used to hearing. Sometimes we need the faith to listen with different ears. Why did my son survive? Why did my best friend's son not? Her son, Bubba visited me in a dream just three days after he died in the tragic accident that threw him from the bed of a pickup truck. His insistent message in the dream was simple. He stood in front of me, looked me in straight in the eye and said three times, "3-4-9. 3-4-9." The third time he was so emphatic that I'll never forget it. "3-4-9!"

A few weeks later, I picked that number, 349, from his mother, my friend Lori, in a benefit lottery and won fifty bucks. Thanks Bubba. But more importantly, I reached for a little book of numbers and meanings by Doreen Virtue and Lynette Brown entitled *Angels Numbers*. The message in their book that corresponded with 349 was this: ***Your purpose involves being an angel on Earth, connecting other people to their Heavenly Source for guidance and support. Ask the angels and ascended masters for their specific guidance and assistance with this mission.*** My purpose of Intuitive Healing Coach was validated with numbers by Bubba from the other side; 349.

The logistics of my life changed very quickly when I returned from North Carolina. I married Chuck, went to Massage Therapy School, and then moved from Pittsburgh to Bradford, Pennsylvania. There we renovated a home that would accommodate a wheelchair, and an intuitive healing room. I would stay the course of *connecting other people to their Heavenly Source* by using my certifications for Massage Therapy, Reiki and Enneagram Life Coaching, offering a healing trio for body, mind and spirit.

Erik and Jenny continue to live their lives in Mebane, North Carolina. I can't imagine how difficult it is for each of them at times, the adjustments and struggles of this unexpected lifestyle. Perhaps that's what fosters the very unique and special bond that has developed between them. Chuck and I took them on a vacation nine months after the accident, to Cabo San Lucas. Way back in ICU, while Erik was in the coma, I kept whispering to him that he couldn't die yet because I had to take him to Cabo and go fishing. I kept my promise. While we were there, Erik asked Jenny to marry him. She said, "Yes."

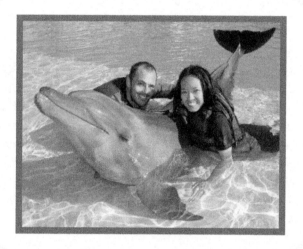

Erik and Jenny in Cabo 2011

Since then, he's been accepted as a participant with the Miami Project Buoniconti Fund to Cure Paralysis in Miami, Florida. He's also been accepted as a potential candidate for an epidural stimulation implant at Frazier Rehabilitation, Louisville, Kentucky in conjunction with The Christopher Reeves Foundation. There are so many organizations committed to helping the paraplegic community. It's a very hopeful time for all of us.

So here we are, at the end of this book, but certainly not the end of the story. Nearly two years ago, I was hoping to reach the hospital in time to say a final *goodbye* to my son before he died. Now I'm hoping that I'll visit the hospital someday to see my son say *hello* to his own child as it enters the world. Jenny and Erik are attempting to conceive by themselves, via electro-ejaculation artificial insemination, at home! They've already had a few takes, and losses, but nothing full-term, yet. I know it's crazy, but true; and it may be the first documented case for this type of homebased conception method.

My son really is something else. And Jenny is more than something else. So as our journey continues, how could I ever give up hope that Erik will walk again, mechanically or naturally? And how could I not believe that he and Jenny have a baby in their future? He has a completely functioning mind and upper body that takes care of his lower body. As he would say, "It really sucks." But it's what he's got and I'll take it, gladly.

I know that Erik is capable of amazing feats. And I also know that the impossible is only possible with God. Even though it's hard at times, I completely trust in the divine plan for his life. Yes, to see my son walk on earth again would be priceless. But regardless, I know he is already walking, in Spirit. Our dreams literally tell us so. And that which makes Erik so very special, his heart, is very much intact.

So who am I to say what's best for my son?

That's between
him and God.

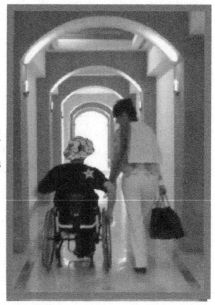

Erik and me in Cabo 2011

the journey continues

Jesus looked at
them and said,

"With man this is
impossible,

but with
God
all things
are possible."

Matthew 19:26

grat·i·tude {noun}

the quality or feeling of being grateful, thankful

& grit {noun}

firmness of character, indomitable spirit

www.GratitudeandGrit.com

Erik's incredible saga continues with the next book,

Paralyzed Without Fear
A Family of Their Own

Mere survival as a paraplegic wasn't miracle
enough; so when the harsh reality of paralysis
turned the dream of having a family together
into a nightmare, Erik and Jenny had to face
their deepest fears and live courageously. They
had more obstacles to surmount, more risks to
take, and more miracles to help create.

Learn more at

www.ParalyzedWithoutFear.com

www.ErikFugunt.com

Made in the USA
Columbia, SC
08 October 2018